Recent Advances in

Surgery

Recent Advances in Surgery 22
Edited by I. Taylor & C. D. Johnson

ISBN 0-443-06191-2
ISSN 0143 8395

NUMBER
23

Recent Advances in

Surgery

Edited by

C. D. Johnson MChir FRCS

Reader and Consultant Surgeon, University Surgical Unit, Southampton
General Hospital, Southampton, UK

I. Taylor MD ChM FRCS

David Patey Professor of Surgery, Royal Free and University College London
Medical School, University College London, London, UK

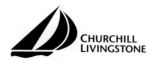

CHURCHILL
LIVINGSTONE

EDINBURGH LONDON NEW YORK PHILADELPHIA ST LOUIS SYDNEY TORONTO 2000

CHURCHILL LIVINGSTONE
An imprint of Harcourt Publishers Limited

First published 2000

ISBN 0-443-064423

ISSN 0143 8395

British Library Cataloguing in Publication Data
A catalogue record for this book is available from the British Library

Library of Congress Cataloging in Publication Data
A catalog record for this book is available from the Library of Congress

Medical knowledge is constantly changing. As new information becomes available, changes in treatment, procedures, equipment and the use of drugs become necessary. The editors and the publishers have, as far as possible, taken care to ensure that the information given in this text is accurate and up to date. However, readers are strongly advised to confirm that the information, especially with regard to drug usage, complies with current legislation and standards of practice.

Commissioning Editor – Laurence Hunter
Project Editor – Michele Staunton
Project Controller – Frances Affleck
Designer – Sarah Cape
Printed in China

Contents

Preface

Welcome to another volume of Recent Advances in Surgery. This book offers specialist reviews and descriptions of current practice in many branches of general surgery, with updates from some of the other surgical specialties. As always, our aim has been to provide an interesting selection, relevant to the needs of trainees preparing for examinations, and attractive to practising general surgeons. We hope this volume will enable you to maintain high standards of practise, and will inform you of developments in areas outside your own specialty interest.

In addition to our regular overviews of advances in general and vascular surgery, we have contributions on sentinel node biopsy in breast cancer, venous disease and a chapter relevant to all surgeons, dealing with possible therapies on the way for the life-threatening conditions of sepsis and SIRS. Specialist areas covered are minimally invasive cardiac surgery, and a unique contribution from Professor Ted Howard on hepatobiliary disease in children, distilling the experience of a lifetime of specialist practice. Gastrointestinal surgery is covered from end to end by chapters dealing with reflux disease, gastric cancer, bariatric surgery, endorectal ultrasound and pilonidal sinus.

We hope that you will enjoy this volume, and we expect you will join us in our appreciation and thanks to all the contributors for their thorough and informative reviews.

Southampton   *C. D. Johnson*
London   *I. Taylor*
2000

Contributors

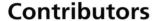

A.M.H. Amin FRCS FRCSG
Senior Registrar and Lecturer, Department of Surgery, Royal Free University College Medical School London, London, UK

Gianni D. Angelini MD MCh FRCS
British Heart Foundation Professor of Cardiac Surgery, Bristol Heart Institute, University of Bristol, Bristol, UK

Prof. J.N. Baxter MD FRACS FRCSE FRCSG
Professor of Surgery, University of Wales, Swansea and Honorary Consultant Surgeon, Morriston Hospital, Swansea, UK

Philip D. Coleridge Smith DM FRCS
Reader in Surgery, Royal Free and University College Medical School, The Middlesex Hospital, London, UK

Neil P.J. Cripps ChM FRCS(Gen) FRCSEd
Consultant Colorectal Surgeon, Department of Coloproctology, Queen Alexandra Hospital, Portsmouth, UK

Peter J. Ell MD PD MSc FRCR FRCP
Professor and Head of Institute of Nuclear Medicine, Royal Free and University College Medical School, University College London, London, UK

Edward R. Howard MS FRCS FRCSE
Professor of Paediatric Hepatobiliary Surgery and Honorary Consultant Surgeon, King's College Hospital, London, UK

Mohammad Bashar Izzat MD MS FRCS(CTh)
Consultant Cardiothoracic Surgeon, Damascus University Cardiovascular Surgical Center, Damascus, Syria

Colin D. Johnson MChir FRCS
Reader in Surgery, University Surgical Unit, Southampton General Hospital, Southampton, UK

Loay S. Kabbani MD
Clinical Fellow in Cardiac Surgery, Damascus University Cardiovascular Surgical Center, Damascus, Syria

Mohammad R.S. Keshtgar BSc MB BS FRCSI FRCS(Gen)
Clinical Lecturer/Surgical Oncologist, Academic Department of Surgery and Institute of Nuclear Medicine, Royal Free and University College Medical School, University College London, London, UK

A. Kumar MS FRCS
Research Registrar, Department of Surgery, University Hospital Nottingham, Nottingham, UK

Lars Lundell MD PhD
Associate Professor, Department of Surgery, Sahlgrenska University Hospital, Gothenburg, Sweden

S.J. Parker BSc FRCS FRCS(Ed)
Surgical Specialist Registrar, Biomedical Sciences, Defence Evaluation and Research Agency, Porton Down, Salisbury, UK

Michael J. Phillips MS FRCS
Consultant Surgeon, Department of Vascular Surgery, Southampton General Hospital, Southampton, UK

J.R. Reynolds DM FRCS
Consultant Surgeon, Department of Surgery, Derby City General Hospital, Derby, UK

Mitsuru Sasako MD PhD
Professor of Surgery, Chief, Gastric Surgery Division, Department of Surgical Oncology, National Cancer Center Hospital, Tokyo, Japan

J.H. Scholefield ChM FRCS
Reader in Surgery, Department of Surgery, University Hospital Nottingham, Nottingham, UK

Asha Senapati PhD FRCS
Consultant Colorectal Surgeon, Department of Coloproctology, Queen Alexandra Hospital, Portsmouth, UK

I. Taylor MD ChM FRCS
Professor of Surgery and Head of Department of Surgery, Royal Free University College Medical School London, London, UK

P.E. Watkins MA VetMB PhD MRCVS
Veterinary Officer, Biomedical Sciences, Defence Evaluation and Research Agency, Porton Down, Salisbury, UK

Lars Lundell

Surgery for reflux oesophagitis and quality of life after fundoplication

The therapeutic aims in the management of gastro-oesophageal reflux disease (GORD) are to achieve symptom relief or resolution and, as a consequence of that, it is assumed that complications to the disease can be prevented. The efficacy of therapy in GORD has traditionally been assessed in terms of symptom control and the efficacy by which the therapy has normalized the endoscopic appearance of the oesophageal mucosa and the amount of acid refluxed as assessed during ambulatory 24 h pH-monitoring.[1,2]

METHODOLOGICAL ASPECTS

Quality of life assessment is a new and important tool to be used in various clinical and scientific fields since the patient's own perceived situation may give important new additive information to the conventional assessment of efficacy variables. Psychosocial factors have a complex relationship with gastrointestinal diseases in general and GORD in particular.[3,4] Existing psychosocial factors, gut physiology and pathophysiology are not associated in a linear, simple or causative fashion, but interact to determine symptoms and illness behaviour. Investigations of similar, potential interactions have received growing attention and involve both hard and soft endpoints. The methodology used and to it related endpoints are those characterized as the physical, psychological status and function and health related quality of life. Health related quality of life is a general measure of outcome from the viewpoint of the patient that includes social and psychological function as well as physical and psychological aspects of performance. The objective assessment of health-related quality of life has become more and more sophisticated as the number of available instruments and potential applications increase. A global, generic and disease-specific quality of life

Prof. Lars Lundell MD PhD, Associate Professor, Department of Surgery, Sahlgrenska University Hospital, S-413 45 Gothenburg, Sweden

instrument may be used alone or in combination and each has advantages and disadvantages.[5] The results of quality of life assessment must be carefully interpreted with the knowledge and consideration of the setting, as well as the potential effects of other factors. Quality of life assessment can never stand on its own or replace other parameters of disease outcome. It has, however, an important impact on gastrointestinal clinical research, since it adds to the available information and has the potential to considerably improve the therapeutic outcome and also to allow the physicians to focus on the clinically relevant issues. For instance, in patient populations lacking objective markers of the disease – such as those with dyspeptic symptoms, post fundoplication symptoms and endoscopy negative reflux disease – it has become more and more apparent that new evaluation tools are required.[6] In GORD where the majority of patients will not have macroscopic mucosal breaks in the squamous epithelium, despite long-standing symptomatology, the application of quality of life instrument allows an accurate assessment of potential problems imposed by these symptoms.

QUALITY OF LIFE IN GORD

Pooled data from clinical studies have shown that general well-being in GORD patients is deteriorated and substantially impaired.[7–10] The level of impairment in health-related quality of life, as assessed by the generic instrument PGWB (psychological general well-being) index is determined by the frequency and intensity of reflux symptoms and is, therefore, consistently lower in patients compared to the reference values. Gastrointestinal symptom clusters are also more pronounced among GORD patients then in the reference group. Importantly, this applies not only to reflux symptoms but also relates to indigestion and other abdominal symptoms such as epigastric pain. Studies have shown that effective treatment normalizes quality of life.

Unfortunately, few studies have addressed the impact of surgical therapy for GORD with particular emphasis on health-related quality of life.

Key point 1
- Gastro-oesophageal reflux disease significantly impairs the patient's health-related quality of life.

QUALITY OF LIFE INSTRUMENTS USED IN GORD

Generic instruments
SF-36 has become one of the most popular and widely used quality of life instruments in the US.[11–13] Population norms with standard deviations have been established to act as standard values in the assessment of individuals or groups of individuals. The psychological general well-being index (PGWB) has been developed to measure subjective well-being or distress.[14] It has been used in a variety of studies on various upper GI-diseases. It assesses six dimensions

of quality of life: anxiety, depressed mood, positive well-being, self-control, general health and vitality.

Disease-specific and gastrointestinal specific instruments

The gastrointestinal symptom rating scale (GSRS) was initially constructed to measure symptom severity in peptic ulcer disease and irritable bowel syndrome.[15,16] It has a 7 grade Likert scale[17] containing 15 items. The gastro-oesophageal reflux disease health related quality of life scale (GORD-HRQL) was designed to assess symptom severity in GORD with particular attention to responsiveness.[18,19]

ANTI-REFLUX SURGERY IN GENERAL

Anti-reflux surgery is designed to improve the function of the gastro-oesophageal junction and to provide GORD-patients with complete relief of all symptoms and complications of reflux disease. Ideally, reconstruction of the physiology of the gastro-oesophageal junction should also permit the patients to swallow normally, belch to relieve distention but hardly to vomit. Data have shown that fundoplication operations restrain the oesophageal sphincter relaxations to water swallows by what seems to be a purely mechanical effect.[20] A major effect of fundoplication operations has been shown to be a substantial reduction in the number of transient lower oesophageal sphincter relaxations.[21] Undoubtedly, these operations also produce a simple, one-way mechanical flap or flutter valve. After the original observation by Nissen[22] that the fundic wrap prevented reflux when studied in patients many years after partial oesophagectomy, fundoplication operations have become the most widely used form of anti-reflux surgery and the efficacy has been established by clinical and endoscopic follow-up and also by use of oesophageal 24 h pH-monitoring, irrespective of whether the operations are performed by an open, conventional technique or by use of modern laparoscopic technology. Over time, a number of modifications to the original fundoplication operations have evolved, but not every surgeon using the actual technique is as satisfied with the clinical outcome as the originator. On compiling data from controlled, clinical trials it can be concluded that obvious clinical differences in the efficacy between different anti-reflux procedures seem not to be prevailing when the outcome is judged with regard to cumulative GORD relapse rate. Excellent control of gastro-oesophageal reflux symptoms can be obtained with a total fundic wrap, a 270° fundoplication, 180° fundoplication provided that each operation involves the reduction of the hiatal hernia couple with the construction of the valve mechanism to re-establish gastro-oesophageal competence. Data are accumulating to show that the outcome after laparoscopic fundoplication is as good as that following open surgery.[23,24] Some failures are, however, unavoidable. Persistent post prandial adverse symptoms can mar an otherwise excellent result in a small, but significant, group of patients after similar procedures.[25–27] The frequency with which these post fundoplication symptoms have been reported varies considerably between series from as low as 0% up to 40%. Dysphagia is frequently reported during the early postoperative period, but vanishes with time as may some post fundoplication symptoms such as bloating and post prandial fullness. Prevention is, however, a primary concern since we lack effective treatment of established severe post fundoplication symptoms. A number of technical considerations have been focused on to counteract some of these problems. There is a wide spread consensus among experienced surgeons that if a complete, 360°, wrap is done, it has to be both floppy and short.[28] Two recent randomized clinical trials have failed to demonstrate any impact on complete gastric fundus mobilization on the short-term functional outcome after a total fundic wrap.[29,30] However, a large randomized clinical trial has reported that a posterior partial fundoplication according to Toupet was associated with less troublesome complains of gas bloat/rectal flatus and also with fewer obstructive complaints in the early postoperative period.[31]

Key point 2

- Effective therapy normalises gastro-oesophageal reflux disease.

SURGICAL THERAPY AND HEALTH-RELATED QUALITY OF LIFE

In 1996, Hunter and his colleagues[32] reported their first 300 laparoscopic anti-reflux procedures and applied quality of life outcome assessments. A significant improvement and normalization in quality of life scores was recorded. By using the SF-36 generic instrument, they demonstrated that surgery improved the quality of life scores in all domains measured by this instrument.

Key point 3

- Surgical therapy effectively and durably controls gastro-oesophageal reflux disease.

A recent study from our unit[33] compared quality of life outcomes of laparoscopic and open anti-reflux procedures. Although not a randomized study, it compared the last 25 open anti-reflux procedures to the first 25 laparoscopic operations done by the group after the learning curve had been passed. All data were retrieved during prospective controlled clinical research conditions. At 6 and 12 months postoperatively, both patient groups had similar scores in the PGWB instruments which reached normal levels (Fig. 1). Using the SF-36 as an outcome measure, another study showed a significant difference at 6 weeks postoperatively in favour of laparoscopic anti-reflux surgery compared to the open approach, primarily in the domains of physical

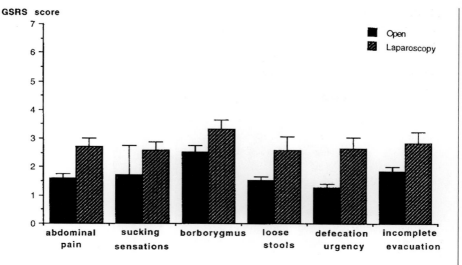

Fig. 1 Quality of life assessed by the disease specific GSRS (gastrointestinal symptom rating scale) after open or laparoscopic operations.[33] The mean and SE are given.

functioning, physical role and vitality.[18] These observations coincide with the generally held view that patients recover more quickly after laparoscopic anti-reflux surgery than after an open procedure. We recently observed that quality of life assessed even 4 weeks after a laparoscopic total fundoplication was significantly improved compared to the pre-operative situation to a level seen in healthy controls (Fig. 2).[30] We also found that – irrespective of whether quality of life was assessed by use of PGWB, GSRS or reflux visual analogue scales – these were stable and at normal levels both at 6 and 12 months postoperatively.[33] With regards to some PGWB items, a slight difference was observed between the open and laparoscopic surgical approach. One possible explanation may be found in the obvious differences in the GSRS. A statistically and significant difference was found between the study groups in symptoms associated with the dyspeptic and bowel dysfunction syndromes (Fig. 1). These differences in GSRS outcomes can, of course, adversely affect the mode level and the self-controlled dimension as well. Two factors have to be considered when explaining these differences in clinical outcome. There are technical and functional differences between various fundoplication procedures. Almost half of the patients included in the open surgical study group had a posterior fundoplication which has been shown to be followed by less post fundoplication complaints of bloating character (primarily rectal flatus). Investigators have sometimes noted a tendency towards a higher frequency of patients complaining of inability to belch after laparoscopic anti-reflux surgery. These observations are worrying as recent data suggest a significantly higher complication rate in the form of obstructive complaints after a laparoscopic compared to an open surgical approach.[34]

Another aspect on the utility of quality of life scales is found in the pre-operative assessment of patients in order to identify those who would react

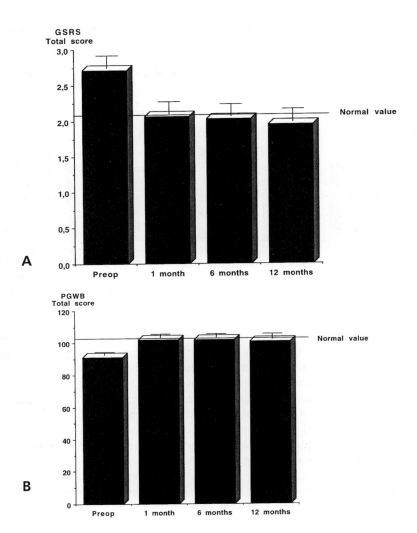

GSRS
Total score

Fig. 2 (**A**) Gastrointestinal symptom rating scale (GSRS). (**B**) PGWB (psychological general well-being) scores in patients assessed during the first year after a laparoscopic fundoplication.[30] The mean and SE are given.

unfavourably to anti-reflux surgery. By use of the GERD HRQL scores, patients were recruited with high pretreatment scores and the subsequent postoperative investigations indicated a high success rate in these patients after anti-reflux surgery. Furthermore, patients who were dissatisfied with the operation tended to have lower pre-operative scores in the mental health domain of the SF-36 instrument showing that GORD symptom relief is a quite complex process and not simply caused by correcting the pathological reflux.[18,19] Studies are needed to clarify the role of these instruments in defining the eventual adverse profile of those who are exposed to high risk of failure after anti-reflux surgery.

Key point 4

- The laparoscopic approach has popularised surgical therapy for gastro-oesophageal reflux disease.

Finally, a special perspective on anti-reflux surgery was gained from a recent randomized, controlled clinical trial comparing omeprazole with open anti-reflux surgery. During a 3 year follow-up period, a significant difference was noted in favour of anti-reflux surgery which also manifested itself in a corresponding difference in the reflux dimension of the GSRS scale.[35] However, due to some gas bloat complaints, an inability to belch and vomit and rectal flatus in the surgical group, other dimensions of the GSRS instrument counteracted this surgical advantage, giving a total GSRS score that did not differ between the two treatment strategies. Similarly, the PGWB score was normalized already 2 months after randomization and initiation of therapy and remained so during the entire study period. These results again emphasize that medical and surgical therapy normalize the impaired quality of life in GORD patients. This unique data base also reiterates the need for further refinement of the surgical procedures with the aim of reconstructing the physiology of the gastro-oesophageal junction without adding postsurgical adverse consequences of functional character.

Key point 5

- The functional outcome after surgery depends on who is doing the operation and what type of anti-reflux procedure is done.

Key points for clinical practice

- Gastro-oesophageal reflux disease significantly impairs the patient's health-related quality of life.

- Effective therapy normalises gastro-oesophageal reflux disease.

- Surgical therapy effectively and durably controls gastro-oesophageal reflux disease.

- The laparoscopic approach has popularised surgical therapy for gastro-oesophageal reflux disease.

- The functional outcome after surgery depends on who is doing the operation and what type of anti-reflux procedure is done.

Recent Advances in Surgery 23

References

1. Lundell L. New information relevant to long term management of endoscopy negative reflux disease. Element Pharmacol Ther 1997; 11 (Suppl 2): 93–98.

2. Armstrong D, Inauen W, Blum A L. Diagnostic assessment of gastro-oesophageal reflux disease: what is possible vs. what is practical? Hepatogastroenterology 1992; 39 (Suppl 1): 3–13.

3. Bradley L A, Richter J E, Pulliam T J et al. The relationship between stress and symptoms of gastroesophageal reflux: the influence of psychological factors. Am Gastroenterol 1993; 88: 11–19.

4. Drossman D A. The role of psychological factors and gastrointestinal illness. Scand J Gastroenterol 1996; 31 (Suppl. 221): 1–4.

5. Dimenäs E, Dahlöf C, Jern S, Wiklund I. Defining quality of lie in medicine. Scand Prim Health Care 1990; Suppl 1 :7–10.

6. Havelund T, Lind T, Wiklund I et al. Quality of life in patients with heartburn but without esophagitis: effects of treatment with omeprazole. Am J Gastroenterol 1999; 94: 1782–1789.

7. Dimenäs E, Glise H, Hallerbäck B, Hernqvist H, Svedlund J, Wiklund I. Quality of life in patients with upper gastrointestinal symptoms. An improved evaluation of treatment regimens. Scand J Gastroenterol 1993; 28: 681–687.

8. Stacey J H, Miocevich M L, Sacks G E. The effect of ranitidine (as effervescent tablets) on the quality of life of GORD patients. Br J Clin Pract 1996; 50: 190–194.

9. Dimenäs E, Glise H, Hallerbäck B, Hernqvist H, Svedlund J, Wiklund I. Well-being and gastrointestinal symptoms among patients referred to endoscopy owing to suspected duodenal ulcer. Scand J Gastroenterol 1995; 30: 1046–1052.

10. Glise H, Hallerbäck B. Quality of life assessments in the evaluation of gastroesophageal reflux and peptic ulcer disease before during and after treatment. Scand J Gastroenterol 1995; 30 (Suppl. 208): 133–135.

11. McHorney C A, Ware Jr J E, Ratczek A E. The MOS 36-item short form health survey (SF-36): II. Psychometric and clinical tests of validity in measuring physical and mental health constructs. Med Care 1993; 31: 247–263.

12. McHorney C A, Konsinski M, Ware J E. Comparisons of the costs and quality of norms for the SF-36 health survey collected by mail vs telephone interview: results from a national survey. Med Care 1994; 6: 551–567.

13. McHorney C A, Ware Jr J E, Lu J F R, Sherbourne C D. The MOS 36-item health survey (SF-36): III. Tests of data quality, scaling assumptions, and reliability across diverse patient groups. Med Care 1994: 32; 40–46.

14. Dupuy H J. Psychological general well-being (PGWB) index. In: Wenger N K, Mattsson M E, Furberg C F, Elinson J. (eds) Assessment of Quality of Life in Clinical Trials of Cardiovascular Therapies. New York: le Jacq Publishing, 1984; 170–183.

15. Svedlund J, Sjödin I, Dotevall G. GSRS – a clinical rating scale for gastrointestinal symptoms in patients with irritable bowel syndrome and peptic ulcer disease. Dig Dis Sci 1988; 33: 129–134.

16. Glise H, Hallerbäck B, Wiklund I. Quality of life: a reflection of symptoms and concerns. Scand J Gastroenterol 1996; 31 (Suppl 221): 14–17.

17. Likert R. A technique for measurements of attitudes. Arch Psychol 1932: 140: 45.

18. Velanovich V, Vallance S R, Gusz J R, Tapia F V, Harkabus M A. Quality of life scale for gastroesophageal reflux disease. J Am Coll Surg 1996; 183: 217–224.

19. Velanovich V, Karmy Jones R. Measuring gastroesophageal reflux disease: relationship between health related quality of life scores and physiologic parameters. Am Surg 1998; 64: 649–653.

20. Stein H J, DeMeester T R, Hinder R A. Outpatient physiologic testing and surgical management of foregut motility disorders. Curr Probl Surg 1992; 29: 415–555.

21. Rydberg L, Ruth M, Lundell L. Mechanism of action of antireflux procedures. Br J Surg 1999; 86: 405–410.

22. Nissen R. Eine einfache Operation zur Be-einflussung der Refluxösophagitis. Schw Med Wochenschr 1956; 86: 590–593.

23. Jamieson G, Watson D, Britten-Jones R, Mitchell P, Anvari M. Laparoscopic Nissen fundoplication. Ann Surg 1994; 2 :137–145.

24. Perdikies G, Hinder R A, Lund R J et al. Laparoscopic Nissen fundoplication: where do

we stand? Surg Laparosc Endosc 1997; 7: 17–21.

25. Negre J B. Postfundoplication symtoms. Do they restrict the success of Nissen fundoplication? Ann Surg 1983; 198: 698–700.

26. Garstin W I, Hohnston G W, Kennedy T L, Spencer E S. Nissen fundoplication: the unhappy 15%. J R Coll Surg Edinb 1986; 31: 207.

27. Spechler J S, Department of Veterans Affairs Gastroesophageal Reflux Disease Study Group. Comparison of medical and surgical therapy for complicated gastro-oesophageal reflux disease in veterans. N Engl J Med 1992; 326: 786–792.

28. Peters J H, DeMeester T R, Crookes P, Oberg S, de Vos Shoop M, Hagen J A, Bremner C G. The treatment of gastroesophageal reflux disease with laparoscopic Nissen fundoplication: prospective evaluation of 100 patients with 'typical' symptoms. Ann Surg 1998; 228: 40–50.

29. Watson D I, Pike E G K, Baigrie J et al. Prospective double blind randomized trial of laparoscopic Nissen fundoplication with diet division and without division of short gastric vessels. Ann Surg 1997; 226: 642–652.

30. Blomqvist A, Dalenbäck J, Hagedorn C et al. The impact of complete gastric fundus mobilization on the outcome after laparoscopic total fundoplication. J Gastrointest Surg 2000: In press.

31. Lundell L, Abrahamsson H, Ruth M, Sandberg N, Olbe L. Lower oesophageal sphincter characteristics and oesophageal acid exposure following partial or 360 fundoplication: results of a prospective randomized clinical study. World J Surg 1991; 15: 115–120.

32. Hunter J G, Trus T L, Branum G D et al. A physiological approach for laparoscopic fundoplication for gastroesophageal reflux disease. Ann Surg 1996; 223: 673–687.

33. Blomqvist A. Lönroth H, Dalenbäck J, Ruth M, Wiklund I, Lundell L. Quality of life assessment after laparoscopic and open fundoplications. Results of a prospective, clinical study. Scand J Gastroenterol 1996; 31: 1052–1058.

34. Bais J E, von Lanschot J J B, Bonjer H J et al. Randomized study comparing laparoscopic and conventional Nissen fundoplication. Patient inclusion ended after inter analysis. Gastroenterology 1999; 116: A117.

35. Lundell L, Dalenbäck J, Hattlebakk J et al. Omeprazole or anti reflux surgery in the long term management of gastroesophageal reflux disease: results of a multicenter, randomized clinical trial. Gastroenterology 1998; 114: A207.

Surgery for reflux oesophagitis and quality of life after fundoplication

Mitsuru Sasako

Surgery for gastric cancer

ADENOCARCINOMA OF THE STOMACH

LYMPH NODE DISSECTION FOR CURABLE ADVANCED TUMOURS

The therapeutic value of lymph node dissection for gastric cancer has been debated in Western countries for several decades, because much better results of surgical treatment for this disease were constantly reported from Japan. A minority of Western surgeons followed the Japanese strategy of extended lymph node dissection and, in the late 1980s, several specialized centres in the West started to report a significant benefit from extended lymphadenectomy over conventional limited resection (even more limited than D_1 dissection).[1-3] These papers reported that postoperative mortality after D_2 dissection did not increase and was 3–5%. However, several papers demonstrated the relevance of the stage migration phenomenon in stage-specific survival rates after extended surgery. Certainly the wider the lymph node dissection, the more accurate the staging, which leads to an apparent increased survival rate for several stages after extended dissection. Bunt demonstrated this phenomenon using the stage-specific survival rates of gastric cancer patients.[4]

A retrospective analysis of a large number of advanced gastric cancer cases showed a high incidence of lymph node metastasis and good prognosis for those having metastasis even to second tier nodes[5] following D_2 dissection (Table 1). In the situation where no alternative therapy can control lymph node metastasis, surgical resection seems to be the only means to control local extension of the disease. This paper showed the benefit of extended dissection without using any stratification by stage, thus circumventing the stage migration phenomenon. The conclusions were not contradicted.

Prof. Mitsuru Sasako MD PhD, Professor of Surgery, Chief, Gastric Surgery Division, Department of Surgical Oncology, National Cancer Center Hospital, 5-1-1, Tsukiji, Chuo-ku, Tokyo 104-0045, Japan

Table 1 Incidence of lymph node metastasis and 5-year survival rates of those having nodal metastasis in each station, according to the tumour location (from Sasako et al[12])

Station	A (distal third)		M (middle third)		C (proximal third)		AMC (entire stomach)	
	Incidence	5YSR	Incidence	5YSR	Incidence	5YSR	Incidence	5YSR
1	6.2	25.0	15.0	52.6	38.0	31.7	32.7	11.3
2	7.1	0.0	3.4	25.0	22.0	23.2	18.2	8.0
3	40.9	42.2	44.8	58.7	45.1	37.9	66.0	17.8
4	34.2	42.3	26.8	48.4	14.5	20.5	53.1	19.0
5	10.5	37.5	2.4	33.3	3.0	0.0	14.2	18.8
6	46.3	46.0	14.6	26.8	6.8	6.3	37.7	18.7
7	23.4	34.9	22.6	46.5	26.9	19.7	44.4	18.5
8	24.5	30.6	11.0	41.5	10.2	20.0	30.6	19.2
9	12.8	30.4	11.0	47.5	16.0	20.5	18.5	20.7
10	3.8	0.0	11.9	33.3	17.4	21.6	21.6	7.4
11	6.7	15.4	6.3	21.4	16.1	11.4	20.6	3.7
12	9.0	29.6	1.6	33.3	2.5	0.0	4.4	0.0
13	8.3	0.0	0.0	0.0	2.5	0.0	5.6	0.0
14	14.6	14.3	8.7	0.0	10.0	0.0	4.5	0.0
16	13.1	18.2	7.4	0.0	12.1	0.0	26.5	11.1

Incidence was calculated by dividing the number of patients with metastasis in each station by the number of patients who underwent dissection of that station. Survival rates of positive patients in each station were calculated irrespective of nodal metastasis to other stations. 5YSR, 5-year survival rate.

In the late 1980s, two randomized controlled trials were started in the UK and The Netherlands, to answer, in a more direct way, the question whether or not an extended lymph node dissection has any therapeutic value for gastric carcinoma. The short-term results of these trials were reported in 1995 by the Dutch group[6] and in 1996 by the British group.[7] Both showed significantly worse results for D_2 dissection: postoperative mortality after D_2 was 10% and 13 %, while that of D_1 was 4% and 6% in the Dutch and British trial, respectively. Morbidity after D_2 was significantly higher than after D_1. Long-term results could not show any significant difference in survival between the two treatment arms.[8] 5-year survival rates of the D_1 and D_2 groups were 45% and 47%, respectively, in the Dutch trial. Disease-free survival rates of the patients who had R0 resection were 57% and 63% after D_1 and D_2 dissection, respectively. In most subset analyses of disease-free survival, the D_2 group had better survival than the D_1 group. The difference in 5-year survival in those patients who did not undergo splenectomy (59% for D_1 and 71% for D_2) and in those who had more than 25 nodes (47% for D_1 and 64% for D_2) was

Key point 1

• D_2 node dissection can improve late survival.

statistically significant. In the same issue of the *New England Journal of Medicine* in which the Dutch results were published, Brennan concluded in the editorial as follows: 'If extended lymph-node dissection can be performed with low rates of morbidity and mortality, then staging will be more accurate and the results of dissection in the West can approximate those in Japan'.[9] In other words, the survival advantage of D_2 dissection over D_1 is estimated as 10–15% in each stage but will become minimal if the postoperative mortality of D_2 exceeds 5–6%.

Key point 2

- In most Western series, the benefit of D_2 dissection is balanced by increased operative morbidity and mortality rates.

These results raised arguments regarding the quality control of surgical treatment in multi-centre clinical trials, especially when a treatment arm is complicated and technically demanding. These two trials had a major difference in the effort of quality control of surgery, while the basic structures of the protocols were similar. In the Dutch trial, a Japanese expert in gastric cancer surgery stayed in The Netherlands for 4 months at the beginning of the trial to teach some of participating surgeons the technique of D_2 dissection.[8] After this instruction period, one of the regional quality controllers attended all D_2 dissections. They learned the technique from the Japanese instructor 1–3 times during the instruction period. Besides this, on-the-job training using 33 operations, a video tape of D_2 dissection which was carried out by the Japanese instructor on a Dutch patient and a booklet explaining the anatomy and the technique for D_2 dissection were distributed to all participating surgeons. Thus, in the instructive period, even the first patient could be randomized. On the other hand, the quality control and instruction of D_2 dissection in the British trial was poor, i.e. distribution of a video tape of D_2 dissection alone. The Dutch trial had better quality control but still the average number of patients per hospital per year was just 1.0, which is too limited an experience to learn the technique and patient management.[10] Further argument for specialization in gastric cancer treatment will be discussed later.

More extensive lymph node dissection is carried out not only in Japan but also in some Western countries. De Manzoni reported the results of 38 patients who underwent a D_4 dissection (defined by the first edition of the *Japanese Classification of Gastric Cancer*[11]). The postoperative mortality was just 3% and 5-year survival rate was 70%, which was significantly better than a contemporary cohort undergoing D_1 dissection in the same department. Although comparison between type of dissection cannot avoid selection bias, the results achieved by the D_4 dissection were still admirable. Retrospective analyses in Japanese patients have shown that the incidence of metastasis to the para-aortic nodes is 20–30% from T3 tumours and the 5-year survival rate of patients who had para-aortic lymph node metastasis was 15–35%. Based on these results, a randomized controlled study, comparing D_2 dissection versus D_2 plus para-aortic node dissection, has been carried out in Japan, starting in

August 1995. This is the first randomized comparative clinical trial on surgical treatment of gastric cancer in Japan. Through the foundation of the Japan Clinical Oncology Group, which has an independent data centre and serves as protocol review committee, monitoring committee, and audit committee, it has become possible to organize a high quality clinical trial. The expected number of patients, about 200 in each arm, will be accrued by the summer of 2000.

COMBINED RESECTION OF ADJACENT ORGANS

Survival benefit from resection of neighbouring organs invaded by the primary tumour has been widely reported.[12,13] Considering the high incidence of distant metastasis from T4 tumours, any T4 tumour which can be treated with curative intent should be regarded as having a good biological nature. If there is no peritoneal seeding, liver metastasis or bulky nodal metastasis, and with negative peritoneal lavage cytology, aggressive resection of directly invaded organs is worthwhile if the surgeon has enough experience of technically demanding operations like Whipple's procedure and subsequent care after such major operations.

On the contrary, the benefit of combined resection to achieve lymph node dissection is doubtful. A pancreas preserving total gastrectomy (PPTG) has become the standard procedure for D_2 total gastrectomy in Japan. In this procedure, the splenic artery is divided at its origin when the dorsal pancreatic artery originates from the celiac artery or after branch-off of the dorsal pancreatic artery in cases where it originated from the splenic artery itself (modified PPTG). All the branches and adipose connective tissue surrounding this artery together with the spleen are dissected *en bloc*, with complete preservation of the pancreatic parenchyma. Maruyama reported the details of this technique.[14] Although this operation is technically more demanding and meticulous than a total gastrectomy with a pancreatico-splenectomy (TGPS), PPTG has much less postoperative morbidity and mortality and as good long-term results as TGPS. In the National Cancer Center Hospital Tokyo, surgical complication occurred after TGPS and PPTG in 39.4% and 19.6% of patients, respectively. Pacelli et al were able to reproduce similar results using a modified PPTG.[15] In their modification, the splenic artery is preserved up to a more distal point.

Further extended resection of uninvolved organs than TGPS is the left upper abdominal evisceration. A few Japanese authors have reported the results of this procedure, but its benefit over conventional D_2 PPTG plus para-aortic node dissection is unclear, because the comparison between them is always historical, and confounded by stage migration.[16]

In both the Dutch and the British trials, the standard operation for advanced cancer of the middle and proximal part was a TGPS. The postoperative morbidity and mortality analyses showed significantly higher risk for those who underwent TGPS than those who did not have combined resection. In the Dutch trial, splenectomy showed a significantly higher risk of operative death (RR = 2.16, 95% CI: 1.09–4.28) and overall morbidity (RR = 2.13, 95% CI: 1.44–3.16). Splenectomy showed a much higher relative risk than D_2 dissection itself.[17] The effect on long-term survival of splenectomy is still unclear. Simple comparisons of patients with or without splenectomy cannot elucidate the effect of splenectomy, because the lesions necessitating splenectomy are usually proximally located and subsequently have worse prognosis than cancers of the distal stomach.[18] Griffith et al reported better survival after gastrectomy without splenectomy than with splenectomy.[19] However, tumour location between the two groups might be quite different because the spleen preserving group included many subtotal gastrectomy cases (98 of 119) while all patients underwent a total gastrectomy in the splenectomy group. Whether the splenectomy itself affects prognosis or not should be studied by randomized trials in the near future.

Key point 3

• There is evidence to favour preservation of the pancreas, and possibly also of the spleen, in total radical gastrectomy.

METHOD OF RECONSTRUCTION

The Dutch and British trials of D1 versus D2 dissection showed high morbidity and mortality for D_2 dissection. In the face of such a high mortality after gastric surgery, the safest reconstruction should be chosen if the quality of life in the long-term is acceptable. The incidence of leakage after gastroduodenostomy, Billroth type 1 (B1), was 2–4% higher than after gastrojejunostomy, Roux-en-Y or Billroth type 2 (B2), nearly 0% at NCCH. In the D_2 group of the Dutch trial, 3 of 16 (18.8%) patients who underwent B1 reconstruction after distal gastrectomy had anastomotic leakage, and two of them died. Similarly 2 of 40 (5.0%) patients who had Roux-en-Y reconstruction and 11 of 149 (7.4%) with B2 reconstruction had anastomotic leakage. All patients who had leakage, except one, died. Considering the high mortality after leakage in Western patients, Roux-en-Y or Billroth type 2 reconstruction is recommended after distal or distal subtotal gastrectomy with D_2 dissection. After a total gastrectomy, the safest method is the Roux-en-Y reconstruction, because the more anastomoses are made the more leakage occurs. Therefore, I strongly recommend this reconstruction for Western surgeons, whose patients are usually older than 70 years and frequently with co-morbidity like ischaemic heart disease.

Key point 4

• Reconstruction should be simple in order to be safe.

On the other hand, due to the increase in the proportion of gastric cancers detected early, many patients now are cured of gastric cancer in Japan. For these patients with a long life expectancy after gastric resection, which type of reconstruction gives the best quality of life or minimum sequelae of gastrectomy is an important issue. Gastrectomy causes two functional disturbances. First, it causes minimization or elimination of a reservoir for food. Second, it causes early transit of food into the intestine. It causes the so-called dumping syndromes in early and late post-prandial phase. There are several papers reporting the results of studies comparing two or three reconstruction methods, but their conclusions are inconsistent.[20–22] We need a well-planned, large clinical trial to answer this question.

SURGICAL TREATMENT OF EARLY GASTRIC CANCER

Several papers from outside of Japan have reported on treating early gastric cancer (EGC). Kim, from Korea, reported that the incidence of lymph node metastasis was 15.7% in EGC and lymph node metastasis was the only significant prognostic factor for EGC.[23] He emphasized the importance of extended lymphadenectomy for EGC, because even for patients who had four or more lymph node metastases, the 5-year survival rate was 77.3% after D_2 dissection. Hayes, from the UK, reported the incidence of lymph node metastasis to be as high as 43% and second tier node metastasis was observed in 3 of 28 (11%) of EGC.[24,25]. D_2 dissection was strongly recommended for EGC. On the other hand, some papers from Japan suggested limited surgery or endoscopic mucosal resection (EMR) for mucosal cancer. At present, it is generally accepted that any treatment which does not involve nodal dissection can be applied, without increase of recurrence, to the following indications: (i) papillary or tubular histology; (ii) macroscopically superficial elevated type (IIa) of 2 cm or less in diameter or macroscopically superficial depressed type (IIc) of 1 cm or less in size; (iii) no ulcerative change in the lesion; and (iv) mucosal cancer.[27] In some institutes such as the NCCH Tokyo, EMR is applied to bigger lesions up to 3 cm of similar characteristics. In the Japanese situation where many mucosal cancers are diagnosed, some lesions are even of a non-invasive type, just like ductal carcinoma *in situ* of the breast often diagnosed in many Western countries. For these lesions, the risk of lymph node metastasis is so low that lymph node dissection should be avoided. On the other hand, submucosal cancer has a much higher incidence of lymph node metastasis and should principally be treated by D_2 dissection. Kitamura analyzed, retrospectively, the patients who underwent a total gastrectomy and concluded that most of EGC can be treated by partial gastrectomy without any combined organ resection.[28]

Key point 5

- Mucosal cancer can be treated by local excisions; submucosal cancer needs D_2 dissection.

SURGERY FOR CARDIA CANCER

In many Western countries, cancer of the proximal stomach, the oeso-phagogastric junction and the lower oesophagus has been increasing. With this increase, classification of tumours arising near the oesophagogastric junction was proposed by the Munich group and widely accepted.[29] There are two commonly used surgical approaches to these tumours, the left thoraco-abdominal approach and the trans-abdominal only approach.[30,31] It is reported that the incidence of mediastinal lymph node metastasis from advanced cancers at the oesophagogastric junction is as high as 30%.[32] Many Japanese surgeons have used a left thoraco-abdominal approach for these tumours to enable a thorough lymph node dissection of the lower mediastinum. However, the 5-year survival rates of those who had mediastinal node metastasis was less than 10%. Partly because of limited treatment effect of lymphadenectomy in the mediastinum for these tumours and partly because of the improved safety of high oesophagojejunostomy without thoracotomy, using staple guns, a thoracotomy is no longer essential for the treatment of cardia cancer. Now, in Japan, a multicentre prospective, randomized, controlled study comparing the transabdominal-only and the thoraco-abdominal approaches is being carried out to evaluate these procedures in terms of morbidity, mortality and survival.

Key point 6

- The best surgical approach for carcinoma of the cardia remains undecided.

SURGERY FOR ELDERLY PATIENTS

In many countries, the average age of gastric cancer patients is increasing due to the growing proportion of aged people and also a remarkable decrease in gastric cancer incidence in the young generation. Therefore, the management of old patients having gastric cancer is becoming an important issue. In The Netherlands, according to Kranenbarg, 27% of newly diagnosed gastric cancer patients are over 80 years old.[33] The following represent the consensus in the literature: (i) the aim of the operation is to achieve R0 resection; (ii) combined resection of neighbouring organs should be avoided; (iii) limited lymphadenectomy is sufficient if R0 is achieved; and (iv) total gastrectomy is to be avoided if R0 resection is possible with partial gastrectomy.

Key point 7

- In the elderly, the smallest resection that removes all tumour should be performed.

SPECIALIZATION OF GASTRIC CANCER SURGERY

Radical gastrectomy aiming at R0 resection is proven to be the best treatment, whether an extended lymph node dissection is carried out or not.[2,8,11,12,16] Until recently, gastrectomy has been regarded as a simple operation and a procedure

Table 2 Summary of D_2 dissection reports

Author	Type of study	Total No. of D_2	No. per hospital per year	Morb. %	Mort. %	Reference
Siewert[41]	Pro. Observ.	1096	14.4	31	5.0 (11)	Br J Surg, 1993
Sue-Ling[42]	Retrospect.	142	14.2	17	5	BMJ, 1993
de Manzoni[11]	Retrospect.	97	13.9	27	3	Br J Surg, 1996
Brennan[43]	Retrospect.	516	51.6	NS	3	Semin Oncol, 1996
Pacelli[44]	Retrospect.	157	15.7	22	4	Br J Surg, 1993
Robertson[45]	RCT	29	7.0	57	3	Ann Surg, 1994
Bonenkamp[6]	RCT	331	1.0	38	10	Lancet, 1995
Cuschieri et al[7]	RCT	200	1.1	46	13	Lancet, 1996
Degiuli[46]	Pro. one arm	191	8.5	21	3	J Clin Oncol, 1998

Pro. Observ., prospective observational study; pro. one arm, prospective one arm trial (phase I/II); RCT, prospective randomised controlled trial (phase III); NS, not stated; Siewert's mortality is 30 (& 90) days mortality, others are hospital mortality. Retrospect., retrospective. Mort., mortality. Morb., morbidity.

for junior surgeons and general surgeons. This had been a widely accepted feeling in the period when ulcer diseases were treated by gastrectomy. However, it is now proven that even a D_2 dissection, which is needed to achieve R0 resection for many advanced gastric cancers, carries much higher risk of morbidity and mortality after gastrectomy, when this type of operation is performed by inexperienced surgeons and/or in inexperienced hospitals.[6,7] The results of the Dutch gastric cancer trial showed clearly that not only the operative experience but also postoperative management and pre-operative patients' selection affect strongly the results of surgical treatment.[17] Now there is almost a consensus that gastrectomy for advanced gastric cancer with curative intent is no longer a procedure for general hospitals with low volume (Table 2).[34] In the near future, only hospitals where more than 20–30 curative gastrectomies are carried out each year should treat gastric cancer patients. Gastric cancer should be regarded as a specialist disease like oesophageal cancer, hepatic hilum cancer or pancreatic cancer.[34,35]

GASTRIC MALIGNANT LYMPHOMA

Several years ago, low grade MALT-type gastric lymphoma was proven to be associated with *Helicobacter pylori* infection and could be cured by the eradication of this bacterium.[36] Now the first choice of treatment for *H. pylori* positive patients is eradication by dual or triple therapy.[37] Although the reported results of surgery with or without postoperative adjuvant chemotherapy for high grade MALT type lymphoma of the stomach was satisfactory for stage I and II patients,[38] radiation therapy with or without chemotherapy showed even better results for similar patients. Now the role of surgery for malignant lymphoma of the stomach is doubtful and new strategies of non-operative treatments are emerging.

Key point 8

- Pre-operative diagnosis may allow non-surgical treatment for gastric lymphoma, and wedge resection of gastric stromal tumours.

SURGERY FOR GASTRIC STROMAL TUMOURS

Among gastric stromal tumours, gastric leiomyosarcoma is one of the most frequent. Prognostic analysis by Koga showed that these tumours can be classified into two types, high grade and low grade. Metastasis from these tumours is most frequently hepatic or peritoneal tumour and the prognosis of those with metastasis is poor. As lymph node metastasis is very rare in incidence and the prognosis of tumours having lymph node metastasis is poor, lymph node dissection is not indicated. If local resection, such as wedge resection, is possible with a clear margin, it is the best treatment for leiomyosarcoma of the stomach.[40] For a large tumour showing intragastric growth, simple gastrectomy is sometimes needed. For high grade tumours, resection is not sufficient but no adjuvant treatment has yet proven to be effective.

Key points for clinical practice

- D_2 node dissection can improve late survival.

- In most Western series, the benefit of D_2 dissection is balanced by increased operative morbidity and mortality rates.

- There is evidence to favour preservation of the pancreas, and possibly also of the spleen, in total radical gastrectomy.

- Reconstruction should be simple in order to be safe.

- Mucosal cancer can be treated by local excisions; submucosal cancer needs D_2 dissection.

- The best surgical approach for carcinoma of the cardia remains undecided.

- In the elderly, the smallest resection that removes all tumour should be performed.

- Pre-operative diagnosis may allow non-surgical treatment for gastric lymphoma, and wedge resection of gastric stromal tumours.

References

1. Jatzko G R, Lisborg P H, Denk H, Klimpfinger M, Stettner H M. A 10-year experience with Japanese-type radical lymph node dissection for gastric cancer outside of Japan. Cancer 1995; 76: 1302–1312.
2. Siewert J R, Böttcher K, Stein H J, Roder J D. Relevant prognostic factors in gastric cancer. Ann Surg 1998; 228: 449–461.
3. Sue-Ling H M. Radical surgery is essential for treating gastric cancer. Eur J Surg Oncol 1994; 20: 179–182.
4. Bunt A M G, Hermans J, Smit V T H B, van de Velde C J H, Fleuren G J, Bruijn J A. Surgical/pathological-stage migration confounds comparisons of gastric cancer survival rates between Japan and western countries. J Clin Oncol 1995; 13: 19–25.
5. Sasako M, McCulloch P, Kinoshita T, Maruyama K. Therapeutic value of lymph node dissection for gastric cancer: a new method of evaluation circumventing the stage migration effect. Br J Surg 1995; 82: 346–351.
6. Bonenkamp J J, Songun I, Hermans J et al. Ramdomised comparison of morbidity after D_1 and D_2 dissection for gastric cancer in 996 Dutch patients. Lancet 1995; 345: 745–748.
7. Cuschieri A, Fayers P, Fielding J et al. Postoperative morbidity and mortality after D_1 and D_2 resections for gastric cancer: preliminary results of the MRC randomised controlled surgical trial. Lancet 1996; 347: 995–999.
8. Bonenkamp J J, Hermans J, Sasako M, van de Velde C J H. Extended lymph-node dissection for gastric cancer. N Engl J Med 1999; 340: 908–914.
9. Brennan M. Lymph-node dissection for gastric cancer. N Engl J Med 1999; 340: 956–957.
10. Parikh D, Johnson M, Chagla L, Lowe D, McCulloch P. D_2 gastrectomy: lessons from a prospective audit of the learning curve. Br J Surg 1996; 83: 1595–1599
11. de Manzoni G, Verlato G, Guglielmi A, Laterza E, Genna M, Cordiano C. Prognostic significance of lymph node dissection in gastric cancer. Br J Surg 1996; 83: 1604–1607.
12. Sasako M, Sano T, Katai H, Maruyama K. Radical surgery. In: Sugimura T, Sasako M. (eds) Gastric Cancer. Oxford: Oxford University Press, 1997; 223–248.
13. Iriyama K, Ohsawa T, Tsuchibashi T et al. Results of combined resection of invaded organs in patients with potentially curable, advanced gastric cancer. Eur J Surg 1994; 160: 27–30.
14. Maruyama K, Sasako M, Kinoshita T et al. Pancreas-preserving total gastrectomy for proximal gastric cancer. World J Surg 1995; 19: 532–536.
15. Pacelli F, Doglietto G B, Alffieri S et al. Avoiding pancreatic necrosis following pancreas-preserving D_3 lymphadenectomy for gastric cancer. Br J Surg 1998; 85: 125–126.
16. Furukawa H, Hiratsuka M, Iwanaga T et al. Extended surgery – left upper abdominal exenteration plus Appleby's method – for type 4 gastric carcinoma. Ann Surg Oncol 1997; 4: 209–214.
17. Sasako M. Risk factors for surgical treatment in the Dutch gastric cancer trial. Br J Surg 1997; 84: 1567–1571.
18. Siewert J R, Böttcher K, Stein H J, Roder J D, Busch R. Problem of proximal third gastric carcinoma. World J Surg 1995; 19: 523–531.
19. Griffith J P, Sue-Ling H, Martin I et al. Preservation of the spleen improves survival after radical surgery for gastric cancer. Gut 1995; 36: 684–690.
20. Fuchs K H, Thiede A, Engemann R, Deltz E, Stremme O, Hamelmann H. Reconstruction of the food passage after total gastrectomy: randomized trial. World J Surg 1995; 19: 698–706.
21. Nakane Y, Okumura S, Akehira K et al. Jejunal pouch reconstruction after total gastrectomy for cancer: a randomized controlled trial. Ann Surg 1995; 222: 27–35.
22. Schwarz A, Büchler M, Usinger K etal. Importance of the duodenal passage and pouch volume after total gastrectomy and reconstruction with the Ulm pouch: prospective randomized clinical study. World J Surg 1996; 20: 60–67.
23. Kim J P, Hur Y S, Yang H K. Lymph node metastasis as a significant prognostic factor in early gastric cancer: analysis of 1136 early gastric cancers. Ann Surg Oncol 1995; 2: 308–313.
24. Hayes N, Karat D, Scott D J, Raimes S A, Griffin M. Radical lymphadenectomy in the management of early gastric cancer. Br J Surg 1996; 83: 1421–1423.
25. Kitamura K, Yamaguchi T, Taniguchi H et al. Analysis of lymph node metastasis in early gastric cancer: rational of limited surgery. J Surg Oncol 1997; 64: 42–47.

26. Ishigami S, Hokita S, Natsugoe S et al. Carcinomatous infiltration into the submucosa as a predictor of lymph node involvement in early gastric cancer. World J Surg 1998; 22: 1056–1060.

27. Aiko T, Sasako M. The new Japanese classification of gastric carcinoma: points to be revised. Gastric Cancer 1998; 1: 25–30.

28. Kitamura K, Yamaguchi T, Okamoto K et al. Total gastrectomy for early gastric cancer. J Surg Oncol 1995; 60: 83–88.

29. Hölscher A H, Bollschweiler E, Siewert JR. Carcinoma of the gastric cardia. Ann Chir Gynaecol 1995; 84: 185–192.

30. Harrison L E, Karpeh M, Brennan M F. Proximal gastric cancers resected via a transabdominal-only approach: results and comparisons to distal adenocarcinoma of the stomach. Ann Surg 1997; 225: 678–685.

31. Takeshita K, Ashikawa T, Tani M et al. Clinicopathologic features of gastric cancer invading the lower esophagus. World J Surg 1994; 18: 428–432.

32. Kodama I, Kofuji K, Yano S et al. Lymph node metastasis and lymphadenectomy for carcinoma in the gastric cardia: clinical experience. Int Surg 1998; 83: 205–209.

33. Kranenbarg E K, van de Velde C J H. Gastric cancer in the elderly. Eur J Surg Oncol 1998; 24: 384–390.

34. Begg C B, Cramer L D, Hoskins W J, Brennan M F. Impact of hospital volume on operative mortality for major cancer surgery. JAMA 1998; 280: 1747–1751.

35. McCulloch P. Should general surgeons treat gastric carcinoma? An audit of practice and results, 1980–1985. Br J Surg 1994; 81: 417–420.

36. Zucca E, Bertoni F, Roggero E et al. Molecular analysis of the progression from *Helicobacter pylori*-associated lymphoid-tissue lymphoma of the stomach. N Engl J Med 1998; 338: 804–810.

37. Logan R P H, Gummett P A, Schaufelberger H D et al. Eradication of *Helicobacter pylori* with clarithromycin and omeprazole. Gut 1994; 35: 323–326.

38. Sano T, Sasako M, Kinoshita T et al. Total gastrectomy for primary gastric lymphoma at stages IE and IIE: a prospective study of fifty cases. Surgery 1997; 121: 501–505.

39. Miller T P, Dahlberg S, Cassady J R et al. Chemotherapy alone with chemotherapy plus radiotherapy for localized intermediate and high grade non-Hodgkin's lymphoma. N Engl J Med 1998; 339: 21–26.

40. Koga H, Ochiai A, Nakanishi Y et al. Re-evaluation of prognostic factors in gastric leiomyosarcoma. Am J Gastroenterol 1995; 90: 1307–1312.

41. Siewert J R, Böttcher K, Roder J D et al. Prognostic relevance of systematic lymph node dissection in gastric carcinoma. Br J Surg 1993; 80: 1015–1018.

42. Sue-Ling H M, Johnston D, Martin I G et al. Gastric cancer: a curable disease in Britain. BMJ 1993; 307: 591–596.

43. Brennan M, Katpeth M S Jr. Surgery for gastric cancer: the American point of view. Semin Oncol 1996; 23: 352–359.

44. Pacelli F, Doglietto G B, Bellantone R et al. Extensive versus limited lymph node dissection for gastric cancer: a comparative study of 320 patients. Br J Surg 1993; 80: 1153–1156.

45. Robertson C S, Chung S C S et al. A prospective randomized trial comparing R1 subtotal gastrectomy with R3 total gastrectomy for antral cancer. Ann Surg 1994; 220: 176–182.

46. Degiuli M, Sasako M, Ponti A, Soldati T, Danese F, Calvo F. Morb idity and mortality after D2 gastrectomy for gastric cancer: results of the Italian Gastric Cancer Study Group prospective multicenter surgical study. J Clin Oncol 1998; 16: 1490–1493.

Michael J. Phillips

CHAPTER 3

Review of vascular surgery

Vascular surgery continues to evolve since its emergence as a sub-speciality within general surgery about 25 years ago. Most vascular procedures in the UK are now undertaken by dedicated practitioners who at least have a special interest in vascular disease. This is reflected in the coverage of emergency cases, with the withdrawal of some general surgeons from vascular on-call and the creation of collaborative schemes involving vascular surgeons in neighbouring hospitals. Some individual units have joined to form specialist vascular units covering a population of 500,000 with 4 or 5 surgeons and 3 vascular interventional radiologists. The advancement of the treatment of vascular disease using complex (and expensive) technologies requires this kind of co-operation and rationalisation to flourish.[1] Although this may result in improved results for the treatment, for example, of ruptured aortic aneurysms and acute limb ischaemia, there may be deleterious effects to 'in house' coverage of vascular emergencies and training in smaller hospitals as well as greater distances for patients to travel. This change in service provision is not unique to vascular surgery and is reflected throughout secondary care, e.g. the Calman-Hine recommendations for cancer treatment, and will probably be re-inforced with the introduction of clinical governance and the National Institute for Clinical Excellence (NICE).

SURGERY FOR ANEURYSM

ENDOVASCULAR AORTIC ANEURYSM REPAIR

The conventional open treatment of abdominal aortic aneurysm (AAA) is now well established and is an effective way of preventing death. The feasibility of

Mr Michael J. Phillips MS FRCS, Consultant Surgeon, Department of Vascular Surgery, E Level, West Wing, Southampton General Hospital, Southampton SO16 6YD, UK

repair of AAA using endovascular techniques continues to be evaluated and has been covered in a previous volume of this series.[2] Many centres world-wide have been evaluating refined repair devices although when, and if, this approach might replace open repair, remains uncertain.

Concerns have been expressed about durability of these grafts, particularly the earlier devices, with reports of continued aneurysm expansion and fatal rupture because of endoleak (incomplete seal of the graft within the aneurysm or back bleeding from lumbar arteries into the sac). Stent fracture and graft folding, resulting in shortening and ultimately graft failure are also reported.[3] At least one endovascular aortic graft has been withdrawn from commercial use because of these problems.

Recent technological developments are:

1. *Thinner (around 19 Fr gauge) delivery systems to overcome narrow and tortuous iliac arteries and ultimately leading to the adoption of a percutaneous approach.*

2. *Self-expanding, thermal stents that have the capacity to adapt to an enlarging neck after initial deployment and proximal stents that can overlie the ostia of the renal and visceral arteries, overcoming the problem of a short aneurysm neck and making the repair of suprarenal aneurysms possible.*

3. *A modular aortic graft system that allows a degree of flexibility in terms of adapting the graft to suit the patient's anatomy*

It is likely that current technical limitations will be overcome over the next 5 years with improved graft design. These developments may result in the application of endovascular repair to ruptured AAA and thoraco-abdominal aortic aneurysm.[4]

Evaluation of the performance and development of endovascular aortic grafting is very important given the current climate of accountability and evidence-based practice. To this end, two important supervisory groups have been set up. The Registry of Endovascular Treatment of Abdominal Aortic Aneurysms (RETA) is a collaboration between UK surgeons and radiologists and reported at the 1998 Vascular Surgical Society Meeting.[5] Since the beginning of 1996, 367 patients having endovascular AAA repair had been registered; 77% had a successful, uncomplicated AAA repair, 21 (6%) required conversion to open repair and 44 a further endovascular procedure. The mortality rate was 7% at 30 days and is comparable to that of open repair; however an improvement in mortality was shown in 1998, suggesting that a learning curve is being followed. At present, the incidence of complications recorded in the registry is too high and it is also too expensive to recommend endovascular repair as the first-line treatment of AAA. A controlled, randomised study of open versus endovascular AAA repair will be required and this has been proposed at a national level through EVAR (Endovascular Aneurysm Repair) and EUROSTAR, a collaboration of European Centres co-ordinated by the European Society for Vascular Surgery. It is clear from early reports that a close collaboration between surgeon and radiologist in the assessment of patients for endovascular repair, as well as in the procedure itself, is necessary for optimal outcomes.[6]

Key point 1

- Endovascular repair of abdominal aortic aneurysms may become established in clinical practice if concerns about durability are resolved.

SMALL ABDOMINAL AORTIC ANEURYSMS

An eagerly awaited study on the management of small abdominal aortic aneurysms was published in *The Lancet* 1998.[7] The national study, co-ordinated by the Vascular Surgical Society of Great Britain and Ireland, aimed to determine whether open surgical repair of AAA of diameter 5.5 cm or less was effective in terms of mortality and morbidity over 5 years. A total of 1090 patients with AAA of such size and aged 60–76 years, usually discovered incidentally, were randomised to undergo surgery or monitoring. The results showed that the mortality of open repair was 5.8% over 30 days and, compared to the mortality rate of the non-operated group, showed that intervention was not of benefit. Of this group, 321 (61%) continued to expand and had undergone surgery by the end of the study. A total of 309 patients died before the end of the trial, about two-thirds from cardiovascular causes. This important study establishes that surgery cannot be recommended to patients with an asymptomatic small AAA and Scott suggests that patients with an AAA of 6 cm or less can be managed conservatively.[8] If the mortality of AAA repair continues to fall with the advancement of endovascular repair, the recommendation from these studies may need to be reconsidered. This would particularly apply to the sub-group of AAA that continue to expand and ultimately require repair, if they can be identified (possibly by genetic or other marker determination), at an early stage.

Key point 2

- Open surgery cannot be recommended for abdominal aortic aneurysms less than 5.5 cm in diameter.

SCREENING FOR ABDOMINAL AORTIC ANEURYSMS

The prevention of AAA rupture, that has an overall mortality of up to 90%, can only be achieved by early detection, since most AAA are asymptomatic up until the time of rupture. Early detection can be achieved by ultrasonographic screening. A number of local studies have demonstrated a survival benefit with screening[9–11] and a large, randomised, controlled study in the South of England, supervised by the Medical Research Council (MASS screening programme), is being undertaken to see if these benefits can be applied nationally. There is currently a debate as to whether screening will be beneficial and obtainable in terms of cost, i.e. the fate of a national screening programme may be decided by political and financial considerations.

ENDOVASCULAR MANAGEMENT OF FALSE ANEURYSMS

False peripheral artery aneurysms caused by trauma or mechanical graft separation at an anastomosis can present a challenge to the vascular surgeon because of limited access and associated soft tissue derangement. Alongside the advances in endovascular aortic repair, prosthetic (Dacron or PTFE) grafts supported by a metal stent have been developed in order to overcome such problems. These stent-grafts can be deployed using a percutaneous technique via the femoral or brachial artery under local anaesthesia, avoiding the morbidity associated with general anaesthesia and the dissection of an open procedure (Figs 1 & 2).[12]

Key point 3

- The scope of endovascular techniques is broadening, and now includes the repair of false aneurysms.

CAROTID ARTERY ANGIOPLASTY

The role of surgery in the treatment of symptomatic carotid artery stenosis is now well established, while that of asymptomatic lesions is still debated, pending the results of a large European study (ACST) that is ongoing.[13] The advancing technical skills that have been acquired through peripheral and coronary artery percutaneous angioplasty have made it possible to treat stenotic and other lesions of the carotid circulation and this method was first described in 1980.[14] The potential benefits of this approach over open surgery are the absence of cranial nerve injuries, the avoidance of general anaesthesia and early discharge from hospital, although open carotid surgery can now be performed safely under local anaesthesia with discharge possible within 48 h of operation. As with open surgery, the concern over periprocedure stroke and cerebral ischaemia secondary to embolisation and thrombosis remains, and has restricted the wide-spread adoption of carotid angioplasty. Currently, there is a lack of data to determine whether balloon angioplasty or primary stenting is required for optimal short and long-term results.[15] The CAVATAS (Carotid and Vertebral Artery Transluminal Angioplasty Study) is an international, randomised study comparing angioplasty with surgery for symptomatic carotid artery disease and is near completion. Early results suggest that the major complications of disabling stroke and death within 30 days of treatment are similar (6.3% for surgery, 6.4% for angioplasty) in both groups. However, the complication rate in the surgery group appears to be higher than that of recently reported series of open surgery from other centres.[16] Restenosis of around 30% after angioplasty and stenting in the coronary and peripheral

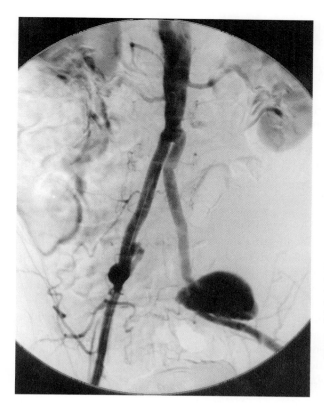

Fig. 1 A false aneurysm at the left graft-iliac anastomosis of an aortobi-iliac graft undertaken 10 years previously. This resulted in a huge retroperitoneal haematoma extending into the thigh.

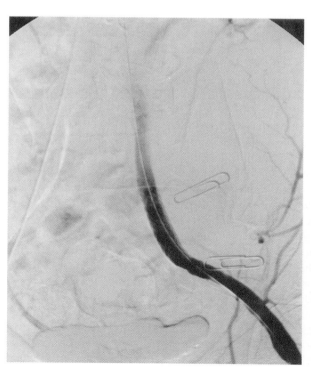

Fig. 2 A 4.8 cm x 10 mm PTFE-covered, balloon–expandable, stent-graft from an ipsilateral groin approach has been deployed across the neck of the false aneurysm and has excluded it.

vascular tree have been the chief drawbacks and the longer term results, i.e. at 1 year and beyond, are awaited with interest.

Key point 4

• Percutaneous carotid artery angioplasty is technically feasible and is currently under evaluation.

VENOUS ULCERATION AND SEPS

Leg ulcers present a significant problem to patients and the health service. They are common (possibly affecting over 1% of the population), painful and disabling. The treatment of ulcers can be difficult and is expensive, costing around £500 million per year in the UK.[17] The recurrence rate after initial healing remains high. The role of vascular surgery in the management of leg ulceration is becoming more established. Many vascular surgeons now have a significant input into hospital and community care; dedicated ulcer clinics have been established and have been shown to be of benefit in the initial assessment and treatment. These clinics can offer clinical evaluation alongside non-invasive investigation with venous and arterial duplex and access to admission for angioplasty, venous and arterial surgery and split skin grafting.[18]

Ulceration is the end result of venous reflux causing chronic venous hypertension. Reflux may originate from superficial veins (about 50%), deep veins (30%) or both. There is available data to suggest that the correction of superficial venous reflux will improve healing rates when combined with compression bandaging in the absence of deep venous reflux.[19] There is uncertainty as to the role of such surgery in the presence of deep venous reflux, although the latter may be improved after the surgical correction of superficial vein abnormalities. Direct surgical correction of deep venous reflux by valvuloplasty, valve transposition and bypass procedures, although theoretically promising, has yet to be proven as an adjunct to ulcer healing. The role of superficial to deep venous communicating (or perforating) veins is also controversial, although there is a well-known association between the presence of lipodermatosclerosis and refluxing perforating veins in the calf.[20] Traditionally, these have been treated surgically by subfascial ligation as described by Linton, Cockett and Rob or by sclerotherapy. The results of surgery are often disappointing, with poor wound healing in the presence of chronic skin changes. Subfascial endoscopic perforator surgery (SEPS) is an attractive approach employing the techniques of minimal access surgery. The major development of SEPS has been undertaken in Germany over the past 10 years and is now beginning to gain interest in the UK, with several instrument companies offering complete packages and there are practical courses available at The Royal College of Surgeons of England in London and elsewhere.

The SEPS procedure (Fig. 3) can be performed under general or regional anaesthesia with or without exsanguination and thigh tourniquet control. A

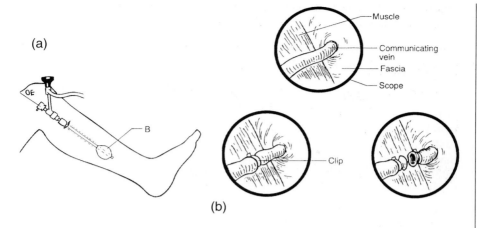

(a)

(b)

Fig. 3 Subfascial endoscopic perforator surgery. (**a**) The operating endoscope (OE) in position with balloon inflated (B). (**b**) The identification, clipping and division of the perforator vein.[26]

small incision is made at the top of the calf, behind the posterior border of the tibia and deepened to the deep fascia, which is then incised. The endoscope is passed down the subfascial space on the surface of the calf muscles with the expansion of this space being facilitated using a balloon. Crossing this space, the perforator vessels can be visualised and divided between vascular clips. Alternatively, they may be diathermied or simply cut. After all identified vessels have been dealt with, the endoscope is removed and the leg bandaged as for varicose vein surgery. A number of preliminary studies have reported good initial results in terms of ulcer healing and a preliminary report of the North American Registry showed 88% healing of active ulcers.[21] Further study is required to determine whether SEPS improves ulcer recurrence rates.

Key point 5

- The role of subfascial ligation in the treatment of venous ulcers is uncertain, but can be achieved by the minimal access technique, subfascial endoscopic perforator surgery (SEPS).

EVIDENCE-BASED MEDICINE AND VASCULAR SURGERY

Evidence-based medicine (EBM) has become fashionable in recent times and is likely to become a feature of medical practice in the future. EBM has its spiritual home at the McMaster University in Ontario, Canada and UK centres have been established in Oxford (at the Nuffield Department of Clinical Medicine) and elsewhere. The Cochrane Collaboration and the York Centre for Review and Dissemination make systematic reviews available, through

> ## Key point 6
>
> • Evidence-based medicine is becoming established and may be applied to the provision and practice of vascular surgery.

printed and electronic media, to anyone with the means of access. Recently, 5 new journals on EBM (e.g. *Bandolier*) have been launched and there are over 5,000 EBM websites.[22] Alongside this upsurge, there has been a negative view that EBM will become a means of further cost cutting and rationing of health care and will be used in clinical governance and health care purchasing. Whatever opinion is afforded, EBM is becoming a powerful tool by which medical practice will be, and is, judged by others.

The Cochrane Collaborative Review Group on Peripheral Vascular Diseases is an excellent source of systematic reviews and is readily accessed through the Internet (http://cochrane.co.uk). It is part of the Cochrane Collaboration and regularly publishes abstracts in the *European Journal of Vascular and Endovascular Surgery* as well as in the *Cochrane Library*.[23] The collaboration is made up of health care workers with a shared interest in EBM, who identify selected information on a subject, preferably involving randomised control trials, from a set search protocol. The information is assimilated and presented as a review. Reviews that are currently available include those on angioplasty versus non-invasive management and lipid-lowering medication for the treatment of intermittent claudication, and the use of patches during carotid endarterectomy.[24] Further reviews, e.g. on thrombolysis, antibiotics in vascular surgery and sclerotherapy, will become available as the Collaboration becomes established.

> ## Key points for clinical practice
>
> • Endovascular repair of abdominal aortic aneurysms may become established in clinical practice if concerns about durability are resolved.
>
> • Open surgery cannot be recommended for abdominal aortic aneurysms less than 5.5 cm in diameter.
>
> • The scope of endovascular techniques is broadening and now includes the repair of false aneurysms.
>
> • Carotid artery angioplasty is technically feasible and is currently under evaluation.
>
> • The role of subfascial ligation in the treatment of venous ulcers is uncertain, but can be achieved by the minimal access technique, subfascial endoscopic perforator surgery (SEPS).
>
> • Evidence-based medicine is becoming established and may be applied to the provision and practice of vascular surgery.

Another source of systematic review of vascular practice is the NHS Centre for Reviews and Dissemination, based at the University of York. A recent publication highlighted the importance of compression therapy in treating venous leg ulcers.[25] For those with access to the Internet, two useful starting points for looking at EBM, are at McMaster University (http://hiru.hirunet.mcmaster.ca/ebm) and at the Turning Research into Practice website (http://www.gwent.nhs.gov.uk/trip) which was created by the Primary Care Clinical Effectiveness Team for Gwent.

References

1. Collins C, Alberti G A, Galasko C et al. Provision of Acute General Hospital Services: Consultation Document. London: Royal College of Surgeons of England, 1998.
2. Dodds S R. Recent advances in the management of arterial disease. In: Johnson CD, Taylor I (eds) Recent Advances in Surgery 21. Edinburgh: Churchill Livingstone, 1998; 147–158.
3. Harris P L, Dimitri S. Predicting failure of endovascular aneurysm repair. Eur J Vasc Endovasc Surg 1999; 17: 1-2.
4. Diethrich E B. Endovascular interventions into the 21st century: what can we anticipate? Eur J Vasc Endovasc Surg 1998; 15: 93–95.
5. Thomas S M, Gaines P A, Beard J D. RETA – The Registry of Endovascular Treatment of Abdominal Aortic Aneurysms. 32nd Annual Conference of the Vascular Surgical Society of Great Britain and Ireland Annual, Hull, November 1998.
6. Beard J D, Gaines P A. The future of vascular surgery. Br J Surg 1993; 80: 185–186.
7. UK Small Aneurysm Trial Participants. Mortality results for randomised controlled trial of early elective surgery or ultrasonographic surveillance for small abdominal aortic aneurysms. Lancet 1998; 352: 1649–1655.
8. Scott R A P, Ashton H A, Lamparelli M J. Fifteen years of experience using 6 cm as criteria for AAA surgery. 32nd Annual Conference of the Vascular Surgical Society of Great Britain and Ireland Annual, Hull, November 1998.
9. Collin J, Araujo L, Walton J, Lindsell D. Oxford screening programme for abdominal aortic aneurysm in men aged 65 to 74 years. Lancet 1988; ii: 613–615.
10. Scott R A P, Ashton H A, Kay D N. Routine ultrasound screening in management of abdominal aortic aneurysm. BMJ 1988; 296: 1709–1710.
11. O'Kelly T J, Heather B P. General practice based population screening for abdominal aortic aneurysms: a pilot study. Br J Surg 1989; 76: 479–480.
12. Razavi M K, Dake M D, Semba C P et al. Percutaneous endoluminal placement of stent-grafts for the treatment of isolated iliac artery aneurysms. Radiology 1995; 197: 801–804.
13. Benavente O, Moher D, Ba Pham. Carotid endarterectomy for asymptomatic carotid stenosis: a meta-analysis. BMJ 1998; 317: 1998.
14. Kerber C S, Cromwell L D, Lehden O L. Catheter dilatation of proximal carotid stenosis during distal bifurcation endarterectomy. Am J Neuroradiol 1980; 1: 348–349.
15. McGuiness C L, Burnand K G. Percutaneous transluminal angioplasty of the internal carotid artery. Br J Surg 1996; 83: 1171–1173.
16. Gaines P A. The durability of carotid angioplasty and stenting. In: Greenhalgh RM (ed) The Durability of Vascular and Endovascular Surgery. London: Saunders, 1999: 95–100.
17. Coleridge-Smith P D. Venous ulcer. Br J Surg 1994; 81: 1404–1405.
18. Scriven J M, Hartsthorne T, Thrust A J et al. Single-visit venous ulcer assessment clinic: the first year. Br J Surg 1997; 84: 334–336.
19. McEnroe C S, O'Donnell T F, Mackey W C. Correlation of clinical findings with venous hemodynamics in 368 patients with chronic venous insufficiency. Am J Surg 1988; 156: 148–152.
20. Ruckley C V, Makhdoomi K R. The venous perforator. Br J Surg 1996; 83: 1492–1493.
21. Gloviczi P, Bergan J J, Menawat S S et al. Safety, feasibility, and early efficacy of subfascial endoscopic perforator surgery (SEPS): a preliminary report from the North American Registry. J Vasc Surg 1997; 25: 94–106.

CHAPTER

3

Recent Advances in Surgery 23

22. Kiley R. Evidence-based medicine on the internet. J R Soc Med 1998; 91: 74–75.
23. Royle E M, Michaels J A, Leng G C. Cochrane Collaborative Review Group on peripheral vascular diseases. Eur J Vasc Endovasc Surg 1998; 16: 1–3.
24. Fowkes F G R. Cochrane Collaborative Review Group on peripheral vascular diseases: review abstracts. Eur J Vasc Endovasc Surg 1998; 16: 273–275.
25. NHS Centre for Reviews and Dissemination. Compression therapy for venous leg ulcers. Effect Health Care 1997; 3: 1–12.
26 Browse N L, Burnand K G, Irvine A T, Wilson N M. Surgical treatment of varicose veins. In: Diseases of the Veins, 2nd edn. London: Arnold, 1999.

Asha Senapati   Neil P.J. Cripps

CHAPTER 4

Pilonidal sinus

In 1985, more than 7,000 patients were admitted to hospital in England with pilonidal sinus,[1] but this is likely to be an underestimate of the prevalence of the condition because of untreated disease in the community. There is a male preponderance of 1.5:1 and it typically occurs in hairy young men. However, this condition may also be seen in women (and occasionally in the elderly) who have very little hair on the lower back.

The term pilonidal sinus originates from the Latin words *nidus* for nest, *pilus* for hair and *sinus* for connections to the skin.[2] Its aetiology is unknown; the theory that it is congenital is largely discounted.[1,3] That it is acquired is supported by its rarity in small children and its similarity to the condition seen between the fingers of barbers, due to repeated contact with hair.[3] In the natal cleft, it is thought that skin follicles are enlarged due to the shearing action of the buttocks. Hair then enters these follicles and infection ensues.[4,5] Alternatively, it is held that hair may penetrate the skin directly. Skin that has been moved to the midline may subsequently develop pilonidal sinuses[6] lending support to the latter theory. It is often easier to treat a condition successfully when its aetiology is clear and it is partly this uncertainty that makes pilonidal sinus disease difficult to treat.

The pathology of this condition is that of chronic sepsis. Epithelial lining of the pits extends for no more than 1–2 mm from the surface, below which chronic abscess cavities may ramify widely, but these are thought to be secondary to the pits, rather than the primary condition. No longer is it considered necessary to excise these widely during surgical treatment. Acute abscesses may occur and usually point or drain spontaneously to one side or the other of the midline.

Miss Asha Senapati PhD FRCS, Consultant Colorectal Surgeon, Department of Coloproctology, Queen Alexandra Hospital, Cosham, Portsmouth PO6 3LY, UK

Mr Neil P. J. Cripps ChM FRCS(Gen) FRCSEd, Consultant Colorectal Surgeon, Department of Coloproctology, Queen Alexandra Hospital, Cosham, Portsmouth PO6 3LY, UK

This disease rarely presents after the age of 40 years.[7] Patients may be asymptomatic, may present with chronic purulent natal cleft discharge or with an acute abscess. Initial treatment depends on the mode of presentation and is most frequently surgical.

TREATMENT

No treatment for the disease is free of problems and the disease is seldom dangerous; thus treatment of asymptomatic disease is seldom warranted. Symptomatic disease may present in three ways: (i) as an acute abscess; (ii) a chronic discharging sinus (sometimes with pain); or (iii) an unhealed midline wound.

ACUTE PILONIDAL ABSCESS

An acute abscess is exquisitely painful, usually presents urgently and requires emergency treatment. Many patients with natal cleft cellulitis are treated with antibiotics by their general practitioner allowing resolution without hospital attendance. However, once a true abscess has developed, drainage is required. It has been traditional to drain these widely and curette the abscess cavity; this is painful and usually requires general anaesthesia. This wound will usually heal but the underlying chronic sepsis will not be abolished due to persistence of the sinuses. It has been suggested that wide excision and laying open may be done acutely, thus treating the underlying disease at the same time, but this results in a large painful midline wound that may take many months to heal; in some cases it may never do so.

Our minimalist approach is simply to drain the pus with a 'stab' wound under local anaesthesia perhaps avoiding hospital admission. Once the acute sepsis has settled and before it can recur, definitive treatment can be offered, with a procedure such as Bascom's technique, within a couple of weeks of draining the abscess. By this time, swelling is considerably reduced and pits which previously may have been invisible may be identified and treated.

Key point 1

• Acute pilonidal abscess should be treated by limited incision and drainage.

CHRONIC PILONIDAL SINUS

Many procedures have been described for the chronic situation, none of which is perfect, judged by the yardsticks of primary healing and recurrence of disease. The ideal treatment would be one in which the surgery is minimal and patients need little time away from work. Surgery that can be done as a day case under local anaesthesia is desirable in these days of diminishing health care resources. An operation which results in rapid healing of the wound, abolition of sepsis and no recurrence of the problem is the ultimate aim.

Table 1 Summary of treatment for pilonidal sinus (Allen Mersh)[1]

Method	Time to healing (days)	Recurrence/failure (%)
Curettage of tract	21–52	3–24
Phenol injection	14–61	0–35
Wide excision and marsupialisation	31–90	1–43
Primary closure	10–50	0–37
Asymmetric closure	8–16	0–5

Although simple shaving and removal of hair may control symptoms without operation,[6] surgery is often required when chronic infection supervenes. Brushing of the pits, a then novel method advocated by Lord,[8,9] may be used in cases with minor disease. Application of phenol to the pits has been used,[10–13] with varying results. However, definitive surgery is often required following failure of these treatments.

Allen-Mersh, in his review article of 1990,[1] describes outcomes after treatment by a number of methods, summarised in Table 1.

A prime requirement of any surgical treatment is the avoidance of major morbidity. In the case of pilonidal disease, the most unpleasant complication (which is also difficult to manage) is a persistently unhealed midline wound, commonly seen after other treatments such as laying open or excision of the primary disease. The exact frequency of this is difficult to determine from the literature, since many reports detail disease recurrence, rather than healing failure.[14,15] However, clinicians who manage this condition regularly are familiar with this vexing situation. Such wounds are often painful, prevent return to normal activity (particularly gainful employment) and usually demand regular nursing and medical attention. These wounds can persist for long periods of time.

In today's financial climate, ambulatory treatments that offer rapid return to full activity, perhaps using local anaesthesia, are preferred to more complex procedures, as long as they are shown to be effective in managing the disease. Such objectives are in keeping with the current requirement to reduce the duration of in-patient hospital stay and treatment costs.[16,17]

Key point 2

- Surgical treatment should be limited in extent to the least necessary to heal the sinus. Surgical procedures that keep the main wound away from the midline are more likely to succeed.

Karydakis technique

Karydakis[18,19] has described a technique of asymmetric natal cleft wound closure (Fig.1). An eccentric, elliptical excision is made with mobilisation of a flap from the medial side of the wound. All sinus tracts are excised completely

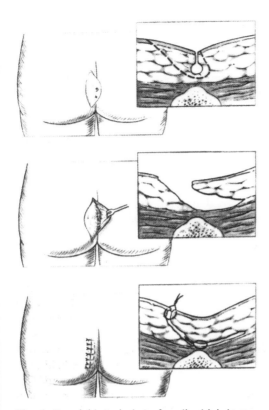

Fig. 1 Karydakis technique for pilonidal sinus.

down to the sacral periosteum. The mobilised flap is sutured to the sacrococcygeal fascia and the wound is closed. The results of this procedure (under general anaesthesia) have been reported in 7,471 patients. The wounds healed well with a recurrence rate of less than 1%, results which have been reproduced by others. Patel et al,[20] using the Karydakis' method, have avoided the situation of an unhealed midline wound, albeit with an in-patient stay of 5 days. Recurrence was not seen but follow-up was not complete. Anyanwu et al[21] treated 28 patients by this technique and reported no recurrences after a median follow-up of 3 years. Primary healing occurred in 88% of cases and all wounds eventually healed. Patients stayed in hospital for an average of 4 days. Kitchen[22] noted a 4% recurrence rate and a slow healing rate of 3%. Mann and Springall[23] have also described an asymmetric excision and primary closure with good results also using general anaesthesia but a mean hospital stay of 16 days.

Bascom's technique
Bascom's technique[4,5,24] is a day-case procedure, undertaken under local anaesthesia, which similarly places the main wound away from the midline (Fig.2). Midline pits are excised removing a minimal amount of tissue (equivalent to a grain of rice) in each case. Care is taken to identify all pits by stretching the post-anal skin caudally; these wounds extend into the 'abscess'

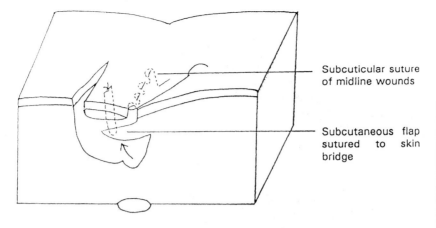

Fig. 2 Bascom technique for pilonidal sinus.

cavity which is then drained laterally to the most convenient side of the midline via an incision parallel to it at a distance of some 2–3 cm. The abscess cavity is curetted, thereby removing all infected granulation tissue and hair. A fibrous and fatty flap (consisting of the lateral wall of the abscess cavity opposite to the lateral drainage incision) is lifted, deep to the midline pits, thus releasing them from the post-sacral fascia. This flap is sutured to the bridge of skin between the midline pits and the lateral drainage wound and the midline wounds are closed with a subcuticular, non-absorbable suture; 4.0 Prolene on a curved, cutting needle is our preferred material. Haemostasis is then secured using mono-polar diathermy.[25]

The lateral drainage wound is neither sutured nor packed and a light dressing is applied to absorb postoperative discharge. All sutures are removed after 1 week and patients are reviewed at weekly intervals until all wounds are healed. Patients are self-caring with no need for attention by a nurse.

It is rare for these wounds not to heal. We have found an average time to healing of 4 weeks. Bascom himself reports an 8% recurrence rate,[4] which is similar to our series of 9.6%[26] and that of Mosquera of 7.3%.[27]

Key point 3

- Karydakis and Bascom have described procedures with greater than 90% success rates.

Bascom's cleft closure technique

A similar procedure to the Karydakis operation was described by Bascom (Fig.3),[24,28] originally for closing the unhealed midline wound (see below). A flap of skin is raised from the least damaged side of the cleft. The underlying sinuses and abscess cavity are curetted and laid open, but are not excised. No

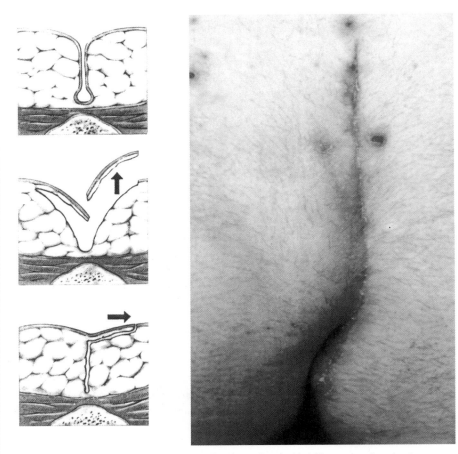

Fig. 3 Bascom cleft closure technique for the unhealed midline wound and primary pilonidal sinus.

fat or muscle is mobilised and the wound lies well outside the sacrococcygeal fascia. The exposed fat is sutured together, thus obliterating the depth of the cleft, and the flap of skin is sutured to the opposite side asymmetrically, having excised sufficient tissue to allow this to lie without tension. This operation is far less extensive a procedure than the Karydakis operation and may be done under local anaesthesia, as a day-case. Wounds usually heal primarily, but, if part of the wound breaks down (often the lower part), it heals rapidly. There are no published results of this cleft closure technique but, so far, we have treated 15 patients for primary pilonidal sinus, some of whom have had prior surgery. The wounds in all patients have healed, although only 33% did so primarily. There have been no recurrences to date.

Key point 4

- Preliminary results suggest that the cleft closure technique may also be effective.

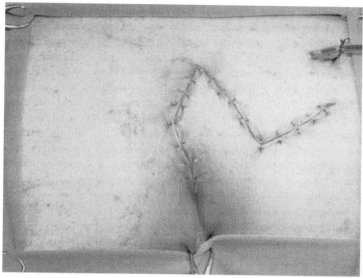

Fig. 4 Rhomboid flap for the treatment of pilonidal sinus.

Rhomboid flaps and Z plasty

Techniques which obliterate the natal cleft are successful in treating chronic pilonidal disease. Tekin[29] has treated 162 patients using a Limberg flap with an average hospital stay of 4 days; 7% did not heal primarily but all healed eventually, although 2% of cases recurred. Azab et al[30] have given the results of 30 rhomboid flaps (Fig.4), with 96% primary healing and no recurrences. Bozkurt and Tezel[31] and Jimenez et al[32] have had similar results and no recurrences.

Z plasty has also been used successfully.[33] Mansoory and Dickson[34] treated 120 patients with no wound disruptions and only two recurrences. Other reports have a high failure rate.[35] A comparison of Z plasty with wide excision and marsupialisation found the former to be superior.[36]

These operations, however, require major surgery and are cosmetically disfiguring. They may be viewed as a 'sledgehammer to crack a nut'; where lesser operations are equally successful, they are probably preferable.

THE UNHEALED MIDLINE WOUND

These wounds are almost entirely iatrogenic and mostly result from the failure of the wounds of excisional surgery for pilonidal sinus disease to heal. The wounds are painful, require regular dressings and result in long periods of time away from normal activity and considerable use of district nurses' time. They are best avoided altogether by techniques described above, but patients unfortunate enough to have such a wound obviously need treatment.

Conventionally, such wounds have been treated with regular dressings, ranging from simple gauze to silastic foam and depilation. Surgical treatment with primary closure usually fails. Cleft closure as described above has been advocated by Bascom for this condition.[28,37] We have undertaken 26 of these procedures for unhealed midline wounds; 34% healed primarily, all have healed and there have been no recurrences of the problem. We believe that surgical correction by this technique should be the first line of management of these wounds and that prolonged periods of wound dressing is an inappropriate use of resource.

Key point 5

- Unhealed midline wounds should be treated by the cleft closure or a flap technique to avoid prolonged changes of dressings.

COMPLICATIONS OF PILONIDAL SINUS

Squamous carcinoma has been reported in chronic pilonidal sinus disease.[38,39] It is, however, rare and does not justify treatment of the asymptomatic patient. Most complications are due to over zealous treatment, which should be avoided where possible.

CONCLUSIONS

Pilonidal sinus disease is a benign condition and patients apparently outgrow its infective complications. It is, therefore, imperative that the treatment is no worse than the disease itself. Prolonged time away from work and unhealed wounds are avoidable. Treatment can now be offered as a day-case without admission to over-committed hospitals. When wounds do not heal, simple surgical techniques exist that can overcome the problem.

Key points for clinical practice

- .Acute pilonidal abscess should be treated by limited incision and drainage.

- Surgical treatment should be limited in extent to the least necessary to heal the sinus. Surgical procedures that keep the main wound away from the midline are more likely to succeed.

- Karydakis and Bascom have described procedures with greater than 90% success rates.

- Preliminary results suggest that the cleft closure technique may also be effective.

- Unhealed midline wounds should be treated by the cleft closure or a flap technique to avoid prolonged changes of dressings.

References

1. Allen-Mersh T G. Pilonidal sinus: finding the right track for treatment. Br J Surg 1990; 77: 123–132.

2. Edwards M H. Pilonidal sinus: a 5-year appraisal of the Millar-Lord treatment. Br J Surg 1977; 64: 867–868.

3. Brearley R. Pilonidal sinus. A new theory of origin. Br J Surg 1955; 43: 62–68.

4. Bascom J. Pilonidal disease: origin from follicles of hairs and results of follicle removal as treatment. Surgery 1980; 87: 567–572.

5. Bascom J. Pilonidal disease: long-term results of follicle removal. Dis Colon Rectum 1983; 26: 800–807.

6. Armstrong J H, Barcia P J. Pilonidal sinus disease. The conservative approach. Arch Surg 1994; 129: 914–917.

7. Clothier P R, Haywood I R. The natural history of the post anal (pilonidal) sinus. Ann R Coll Surg Engl 1984; 66: 201–203.

8. Lord P H. Pilonidal sinus: a simple treatment. Br J Surg 1965; 52: 298–300.

9. Kobel T. Sacrococcygeal pilonidal sinus: is Lord's procedure safe and useful? Coloproctology 1988; 10: 102.

10. Blumberg N A. Pilonidal sinus treated by conservative surgery and the local application of phenol. S Afr J Surg 1978; 16: 245–247.

11. Maurice B A. A conservative treatment of pilonidal sinus. Br J Surg 1964; 51: 510–512.

12. Stansby G. Phenol treatment of pilonidal sinuses of the natal cleft. Br J Surg 1989; 76: 729–730.

13. Kelly S B, Graham W J. Treatment of pilonidal sinus by phenol injection. Ulster Med J 1989; 58: 56–59.

14. Bissett I P, Isbister W H. The management of patients with pilonidal disease – a comparative study. Aust N Z J Surg 1987; 57: 939–942.

15. McLaren C A. Partial closure and other techniques in pilonidal surgery: an assessment of 157 cases. Br J Surg 1984; 71: 561–562.

16. Guidelines for Day Case Surgery. London: The Royal College of Surgeons of England Working Party, 1992.

17. Thompson-Fawcett M W, Cook T A, Baigrie R J, Mortensen N J McC. What patients think of day-surgery proctology. Br J Surg 1998; 85: 1388.

18. Karydakis G E. New approach to the problem of pilonidal sinus. Lancet 1973; ii: 1414–1415.

19. Karydakis G E. Easy and successful treatment of pilonidal sinus after explanation of its causative process. Aust N Z J Surg 1992; 62: 385–389.

20. Patel H, Lee M, Bloom I, Allen-Mersh T G. Prolonged delay in healing after surgical treatment of pilonidal sinus is avoidable. Colorectal Dis 1999; 1: 107–110.

21. Anyanwu A C, Hossain S, Williams A, Montgomery A C. Karydakis operation for sacrococcygeal pilonidal sinus disease: experience in a district general hospital. Ann R Coll Surg Engl 1998; 80: 197–199.

22. Kitchen P R. Pilonidal sinus: experience with the Karydakis flap. Br J Surg 1996; 83: 1452–1455.

23. Mann C V,.Springall R. 'D' excision for sacrococcygeal pilonidal sinus disease. J R Soc Med 1987; 80: 292–295.

24. Bascom J. Pilonidal sinus. In: Current Therapy in Colon and Rectal Surgery. New York: Dekker, 1990; 32–39.

25. Senapati A. Pilonidal sinus. Postgrad Surg 1996; 6: 19–24.

26. Senapati A, Cripps N P J, Thompson M R. Bascom's operation in the day-surgical management of symptomatic pilonidal sinus. Br J Surg 2000. In press.

27. Mosquera D A, Quayle J B. Bascom's operation for pilonidal sinus. J R Soc Med 1995; 88: 45P–46P.

28. Bascom J U. Pilonidal sinus. Curr Pract Surg 1994; 6: 175–180.

29. Tekin A. Pilonidal sinus: experience with the Limberg flap. Colorect Dis 1999; 1: 29–33.

30. Azab A S, Kamal M S, Saad R A, Abou A K, Ali N A. Radical cure of pilonidal sinus by a transposition rhomboid flap. Br J Surg 1984; 71: 154–155.

31. Bozkurt M K, Tezel E. Management of pilonidal sinus with the Limberg flap. Dis Colon Rectum 1998; 41: 775–777.

32. Jimenez R C, Alcalde M, Martin F, Pulido A, Rico P. Treatment of pilonidal sinus by excision and rhomboid flap. Int J Colorect Dis 1990; 5: 200–202.

33. Toubanakis G. Treatment of pilonidal sinus disease with the Z-plasty procedure (modified). Am Surg 1986; 52: 611–612.

34. Mansoory A, Dickson D. Z-plasty for treatment of disease of the pilonidal sinus. Surg Gynecol Obstet 1982; 155: 409–411.

35. Morrison P D. Is Z-plasty closure reasonable in pilonidal disease? Ir J Med Sci 1985; 154: 110–112.

36. Hodgson W J, Greenstein R J. A comparative study between Z-plasty and incision and drainage or excision with marsupialization for pilonidal sinuses. Surg Gynecol Obstet 1981; 153: 842–844.

37. Bascom J U. Repeat pilonidal operations. Am J Surg 1987; 154: 118–122.

38. Abboud B, Ingea H. Recurrent squamous-cell carcinoma arising in sacrococcygeal pilonidal sinus tract: report of a case and review of the literature. Dis Colon Rectum 1999; 42: 525–528.

39. Jeddy T A, Vowles R H, Southam J A. Squamous cell carcinoma in a chronic pilonidal sinus. Br J Clin Pract 1994; 48: 160–161.

A. Kumar J. R. Reynolds J. H. Scholefield

Endorectal ultrasound in rectal cancer

Endorectal ultrasonography (ERUS) has revolutionised the management of rectal cancer. Accurate pre-operative staging of rectal cancer is increasingly being emphasised as it benefits patients in terms of both oncological and functional outcomes. In most of Europe, adjuvant pre-operative high dose short-term radiotherapy (25 Gy in 5 fractions over 5 days) is increasingly being used for patients with resectable rectal cancer as it has been shown to reduce the local recurrence rate (from 27% to 11%) and to improve 5 year survival by 10%.[1] This dose of 25 Gy in 5 fractions is considered necessary to kill microscopic collections of cancer cells in the pelvis. However, there has been concern about the deleterious effects of such a radiation regimen on bowel function in the long-term and about its effect on sphincter function and pudendal neuropathy.[2] Moreover, there is good evidence that surgery alone may be adequate treatment for early rectal cancer.[3] Therefore, it is important to stage rectal cancer pre-operatively and select patients who would benefit from such an adjuvant treatment. ERUS may also influence the choice of operation by identifying early cases of rectal cancer, involving mucosa or submucosa only, which may be considered for techniques of local excision such as trans-anal endoscopic microsurgery (TEMS).[4,5] In addition, pre-operative staging using ERUS may provide useful prognostic information by accurately assessing depth of invasion of the tumour and involvement of mesorectal lymph nodes, the two most important prognostic factors.[6,7]

Endorectal ultrasonography has evolved into a powerful tool for pre-operative staging of rectal cancer. A number of studies, over more than a

Mr A. Kumar MS FRCS, Research Registrar, Department of Surgery, University Hospital Nottingham, Nottingham NG7 2UH, UK (correspondence)

Mr J.R. Reynolds DM FRCS, Consultant Surgeon, Department of Surgery, Derby City General Hospital, Derby DE22 3NE, UK

Mr J.H. Scholefield ChM FRCS, Reader in Surgery, Department of Surgery, University Hospital Nottingham, Nottingham NG7 2UH, UK

decade, have reported its effectiveness in staging primary rectal cancer.[8–13] ERUS has a number of advantages over other techniques – such as digital examination, computed tomography (CT) and magnetic resonance imaging (MRI) – for assessing rectal cancer. The accuracy of digital examination is highly subjective and varies from 60–80%. It has limitations in assessing lesions cephalad to the lower third of the rectum and in determining the involvement of mesorectal lymph nodes. Similarly, CT and MRI are not as accurate as endorectal ultrasonography in assessing depth of local invasion and mesorectal lymph nodes.[9,14–16] CT and MRI may detect extension of the tumour beyond rectal wall or the involvement of adjacent structures, but they do not provide precise delineation of rectal wall structure, including the different wall layers.[15] Positron emission tomography (PET) and radioimmunoscintigraphy provide a functional image rather than precise anatomical definition. At present, there is no evidence for a role for PET or radioimmunoscintigraphy in pre-operative staging of primary rectal cancer.

Endorectal ultrasonography is also useful to identify patients with locally advanced disease, who should be considered for primary radiotherapy to down-stage the disease. Pre-operative radiotherapy appears to reduce local recurrence in this group particularly. ERUS has also been used to follow patients who have undergone sphincter saving rectal resection to detect pre-symptomatic local recurrence.[11,17,18]

EQUIPMENT AND EXAMINATION TECHNIQUE

There are a number of manufacturers of endorectal sonographic equipment and a variety of transducer frequencies and designs in use. The most widely used transducers are 7 and 10 MHz and have focal lengths of 2–5 cm and 1–4 cm, respectively (Fig. 1). Resolution may be improved by increasing the frequency of the ultrasound but this is at the expense of reduced depth of penetration. The longer focal length provides an advantage in examining perirectal structures. The endosonographic transducer is fitted to the end of a rod, which rotates mechanically at a rate of 4–6 cycles/s. The ultrasound signal is transmitted and received at 90° to the axis of the transducer, and this system provides a 360° display of the rectum and surroundings tissues. A latex balloon filled with 20–40 ml of de-gassed water over the transducer is used in the rectum to provide acoustic coupling (Fig. 2). Although the radial probe design is generally regarded as optimal, some authors have used linear probes.

ERUS images are degraded by the presence of air bubbles in the balloon and by faeces in the rectum. It is, therefore, important to eliminate air from the balloon and advisable to administer an enema before ERUS examination.

PATIENT POSITION

Either the left lateral position or lithotomy position can be used; the left lateral is most commonly used for unsedated patients, but lithotomy is the usual position for examination under anaesthesia for anxious patients, or when ultrasound guided biopsy is required. The position in which the examination is carried out affects the orientation of the static images produced and should be made clear on such images.

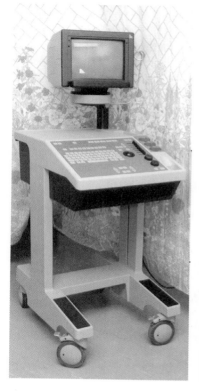

Fig. 1 Cheetah ultrasound scanner type 2003 (B&K Medical).

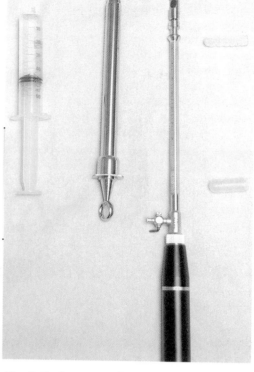

Fig. 2 Equipment used in endorectal ultrasonography. From left to right: syringe filled with de-gassed water used to fill the balloon, sigmoidoscope, endoprobe consisting of rotating rod, overtube, transducer at tip and latex balloon (top right). Also shown at bottom right is plastic cone used for endo-anal examination.

EXAMINATION

A careful digital examination is carried out, palpating the area of interest. A 20 cm sigmoidoscope is then passed into the rectum, the lesion is inspected and the distance from the anal verge is recorded. The assembled endoprobe is then passed through the sigmoidoscope to a position above the lesion. It is possible to reach 20 cm above the anal verge in this way. The endoprobe may be passed blindly for very low lesions. Following insertion of the probe to the end of the 20 cm sigmoidoscope, the latex balloon is filled with de-gassed water. The probe and sigmoidoscope are then simultaneously withdrawn slowly and the transducer is activated so that a 360° scan of the rectal wall and the surrounding tissues is displayed on the screen. The probe can be moved gently backwards and forwards past areas of interest, and the volume of water in the balloon can be adjusted to bring a particular feature into the optimal focal range of the transducer. For most purposes, the transducer should be positioned centrally in the lumen. Video recording of the examination provides a useful record for later discussion.

Two problems may be encountered when performing endorectal sono-graphy. High lesions may be difficult to examine, since manoeuvring of the probe through the lesion may be extremely difficult and there is a potential risk of perforation. Secondly, very stenotic lesions with a lumen of less than 25 mm may also prove difficult, since the balloon is badly distorted and the trans-ducer may snag.

The probe should be cleaned with spirit between cases. If it is contaminated and after use, it should be disassembled and soaked in glutaraldehyde for 30 minutes.

SONOGRAPHIC ANATOMY OF THE RECTUM

In the evolution of ERUS, controversy has surrounded the interpretation of sonographic images of the rectum. However, following anatomical studies, it is now accepted that the five basic layers of the rectal wall seen on ERUS compare directly to the anatomical layers present in the rectal wall. The five layers working from the lumen of the rectum are:

1. *The first hyper-echoic layer is the interface between the water/balloon and mucosal surface.*

2. *The first hypo-echoic layer is the combined layer produced by mucosa and muscularis mucosae.*

3. *The second hyper-echoic layer is the submucosa.*

4. *The second hypo-echoic layer is the muscularis propria.*

5. *The third hyper-echoic layer is the interface between the muscularis propria and perirectal fat or the serosa.*

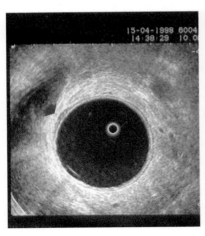 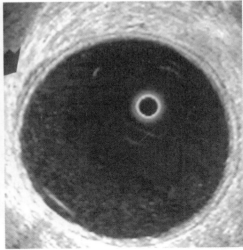

Fig. 3 An endosonogram demonstrating the five layers of the rectal wall, more clear at the 10 o'clock position as shown by arrow. The patient's anterior is at the 12 o'clock position and the patient's left is to the right side of the scan.

This five layered system of interpretation (Fig. 3) is now recognised as the standard for routine clinical rectal sonography.

Some studies[5] have further subdivided the second hypo-echoic layer into three layers, which are: two hypo-echoic layers representing the inner circular and outer longitudinal muscle layers; and an intervening hyper-echoic layer due to the inter muscular layer space.

The perirectal fat has a mixed appearance on the ERUS; since this tissue is mainly fat, it is generally slightly hypo-echoic. Metastatic perirectal lymph nodes appear as oval echo-poor lesions in the mesorectum. In men, the urinary bladder, seminal vesicles, prostate and the bulbous urethra form the anterior relations, while in women the vagina separated from the rectum by the recto-vaginal septum forms the anterior relationship of the rectum. The uterus and ovaries can also be imaged in female patients.

CLINICAL APPLICATIONS

The aims of clinical evaluation are summarised in Table 1.

Table 1   Clinical applications

1. To stage rectal cancer pre-operatively in order to select patients suitable for pre-operative adjuvant radiotherapy, local excision of cancer (TEMS) and get useful information on prognosis.

2. To detect distal intramural spread which may help in selecting appropriate surgery in patients with low rectal cancer located within 6 cm from anal verge.

3. To identify locally advanced cancer cases (T4 lesions) who would benefit from primary pre-operative radiotherapy to down stage the disease.

4. To follow-up patients who have undergone sphincter saving rectal resection to try and detect pre symptomatic local recurrence and to allow ultrasound guided needle biopsies in cases where it is difficult to differentiate between recurrence and fibrosis.

5. To detect malignant change within the rectal villous lesions, guiding appropriate surgical approach.

6. To get more information on extra-rectal tumours like leiomyosarcomas and rare tumours such as carcinoids.

ASSESSMENT OF DEPTH OF INVASION

Endorectal ultrasonic staging of rectal cancer corresponds to the TNM classification, as all anatomical layers of the rectum can be imaged. The letter 'u' is used to indicate an ultrasonic staging:

1. **Tu1** – *tumour confined to submucosa with intact bright middle hyper-echoic layer (Fig. 4).*

2. **Tu2** – *tumour invading muscularis propria with no disruption of the third hyper-echoic layer.*

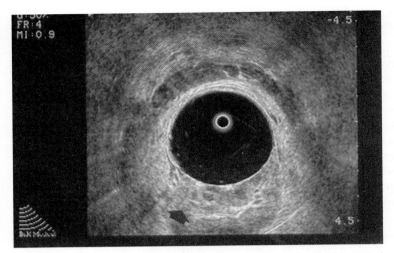

Fig. 4 An endosonogram demonstrating a T1 lesion as the third hyperechoic layer (arrow) is intact.

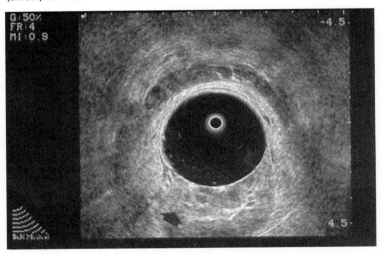

Fig. 5 An endosonogram of a T3 lesion . Here the fifth hyperechoic layer (arrow) representing the interface between muscularis propria and perirectal fat is breached.

3. ***Tu3*** – *tumour penetrating through the muscularis propria (transmural) to invade the peri rectal fat. The tumour edge is usually irregular with saw-tooth projection disrupting the third hyper-echoic layer (Fig. 5).*

4. ***Tu4*** – *tumour invading an adjacent structure.*

Endorectal ultrasonography is currently the best method for pre-operative assessment of the depth of infiltration of rectal cancer, although it is least accurate for T2 and T4 tumours. A meta-analysis of 11 studies found that sensitivity of ERUS was affected by tumour stage, with sensitivities of 84%, 76%, 96% and 76% for stages T1–T4, respectively.[19] Most of the studies[10,13,20–22] have reported the accuracy rates of ERUS in evaluation of rectal tumour invasion to be 67–95% (Table 2).

Table 2 Accuracy of endosonography in predicting depth of invasion of **primary rectal cancer**

Studies	Year	No. of patients	Accuracy (%)
Beynon[38]	1989	100	93
Rifkin et al[29]	1989	102	67
Waizer et al[16]	1989	68	76
Glaser et al[8]	1990	86	88
Tio et al[12]	1991	61	80
Lindmark et al[31]	1992	53	81
Tarroni et al[13]	1992	214	94
Milsom et al[30]	1992	67	95
Katsura et al[10]	1992	120	92
Herzog et al[15]	1993	118	89
Sailer et al[20]	1997	154	78
Akasu et al[21]	1997	164	82

It is known that distal intramural spread, up to 50 mm, can occur in 12–26% of cases of rectal cancer. Assessment of distal intramural spread is important to obtain a clear margin and may be helpful for selecting the appropriate operation in patients with low rectal cancer located within 6 cm of the anal verge. ERUS has been shown to be useful for detecting distal intramural spread > 5 mm in patients with low rectal carcinoma.[23]

Using ERUS, it may be difficult to differentiate between an adenoma and a very early cancer involving only mucosa. Approximately 10% of villous adenomas harbour malignancy that is not clinically apparent and is frequently missed on random endoscopic biopsies.[24] Pre-therapeutic ERUS could decrease this risk by detecting invasion of the muscularis propria and perirectal lymph nodes, the two main contra-indications to local treatment. Sometimes malignant change within an adenoma can be picked up by detecting echo-poor spots within the homogenous pattern of an adenoma,[8] allowing for definitive one stage treatment without risk of tumour transgression during excisional biopsy.

There are many potential clinico-pathological causes of error in rectal cancer staging using ERUS.[21] Some of them are avoidable, hence an awareness of the limitations and pitfalls of ERUS may allow improvement of staging accuracy and contribute to optimum clinical decision making. The over-staging of tumour invasion is mostly caused by tumour invasion close to the deeper uninvolved layer, inflammatory cell aggregation, desmoplastic changes and hypervascularity around the tumour mimicking tumour invasion on ERUS. This is because the echogenicity of tumour is similar to that of muscularis propria and inflammatory infiltrate. Taking a biopsy can induce inflammation in the tumour, resulting in somewhat lower staging accuracy. Under-staging is mostly the result of microscopic invasion beyond the estimated layers, which cannot be detected by ERUS. Other factors, which lead to inaccurate assessment of tumour invasion, are listed in Table 3.

Table 3 Factors which lead to inaccurate assessment of tumour invasion

- Difficulties in endosonographic examination in situations where the tumour is close to the anal canal or the tumour is adjacent to one of the valves of Houston.[21]

- Polypoidal lesions and bulky tumours, which do not lie within the focal length of the transducer, can also lead to misinterpretation.

- Angulation of the probe to the tumour axis can also cause misinterpretation as the obtained images are blurred.

- Radiotherapy can significantly hamper the assessment of wall invasion by ERUS.[25] This is probably because, after irradiation, the rectal wall is thickened, more hypo-echoic and the different layers are less clearly visualized. In these patients, over-staging is more of a problem than under-staging.

- Rectal anatomy may influence staging accuracy in the lower rectum because the structure of the ampulla recti renders endosonographic examination more difficult. In addition, endosonographic layers are less well defined at this level. On the other hand, tumour position with respect to rectal circumference does not influence the predictive value of ERUS.[20]

LYMPH NODE ASSESSMENT

Metastatic involvement of the mesorectal lymph nodes is a major independent prognostic factor. It has been observed that the presence of more than three nodes are associated with poor prognosis.[7] Identification of a metastatic perirectal lymph node is important, as these patients may benefit from pre-operative adjuvant radiotherapy and T1 or T2 lesions with mesorectal node involvement are not suitable for local excision. The detection of lateral lymphatic involvement is equally important, as lateral spread has been noted in the absence of mesorectal involvement, the spread having skipped the mesorectum.[26] Such patients with lateral spread would require wide lateral clearance as extension of tumour to the lateral margin is related directly to recurrence.[27]

The involved nodes appear as circular or oval, echo-poor lesions in the mesorectum. Many other parameters concerning the internal structure of the node have been described in the literature, these are: (i) lobulation; (ii) inhomogeneity; (iii) border delineation; (iv) presence of echo-poor rim; (v) presence of peri-nodal halo; and (vi) presence of hilar reflection. Most of the in vitro studies[28] show that three ultrasonographic features of a lymph node significantly predict its histological status on histopathological examination: (i) short axis diameter; (ii) degree of inhomogeneity; and (iii) absence of a hilar reflection. If a whole node is replaced by tumour or the node is enlarged secondary to it, detection is more likely. However, if only a small deposit or a micrometastasis is present in a node, the characteristics of the node are unlikely to be sufficiently altered to allow detection. Some studies[29] have considered any visualised lymph node adjacent to an area of tumour to be involved. The accuracy of ERUS in assessing lymph node involvement has been shown to be in the range of 62–84% in different series (Table 4). Over-staging and under-staging can occur during assessment of lymph node involvement. Over-staging in node status is mostly caused by reactive lymph

Table 4 Accuracy of endosonography in predicting lymph node involvement

Studies	Year	No. of patients	Accuracy (%)
Beynon[38]	1989	95	83
Rifkin et al[29]	1989	102	81
Glaser et al[8]	1990	73	79
Hildebrandt et al[39,40]	1990	113	79
Tio et al[12]	1991	61	62
Tarroni et al[13]	1992	214	84
Lindmark et al[31]	1992	53	81
Katsura et al[10]	1992	98	
Herzog et al[15]	1993	111	80
Akasu et al[21]	1997	117	77

node swelling and under-staging by the presence of small involved nodes and metastasis in extra-mesorectal nodes.[21] A few reports have described the feasibility and safety of needle biopsy of perirectal lymph nodes under ERUS guidance with a sensitivity of 71% and specificity of 89%.[11,30] In some cases, Doppler ultrasonography may be helpful in discriminating between enlarged lymph nodes and blood vessels.[31] The use of the most effective parameters or better access to regional lymph nodes or a combination of these approaches may lead to further improvement of the staging accuracy.

The published data[14,32] support the notion that ERUS is superior to CT or MRI in assessing perirectal lymph node involvement, although such an assessment requires much greater operator experience than assessment of tumour infiltration in the bowel wall. Imaging techniques such as CT and MRI can demonstrate enlarged lymph nodes but do not allow tissue differentiation within the node.[33] The size of the lymph node itself is not an important factor as it could be influenced by a benign inflammatory process within the node. Moreover, very small nodes (< 5 mm) detected by ERUS and not picked up by CT or MRI might have metastatic disease in up to 18% of cases.[10] Lymphoscintigraphic studies for prediction of nodal involvement have been disappointing[34] and monoclonal immunoscintigraphy remains an investigative tool, as it has not been used for the diagnosis of primary rectal carcinoma.[35]

THE DETECTION OF LOCAL RECURRENCE

Reviewing the literature shows huge variation in the local recurrence rates of rectal cancer ranging from 4% to 32% with a median of over 15%.[36] The causes of local recurrence are many, and include positive histological margins, implantation of viable cancer cells at the time of surgery and incomplete excision of mesorectum. Most local recurrences begin outside the bowel lumen and, by the time they become symptomatic or intra-luminal, they are fixed and, therefore, unresectable. It may, therefore, be useful to identify small extra-rectal recurrence before there is any evidence of luminal recurrence so that a second attempt at curative surgery can be made. ERUS has been shown to be

Endorectal ultrasound in rectal cancer

an effective tool in detecting extra-rectal recurrence by a few authors.[30,37,38] ERUS is especially useful in follow-up of rectal cancer patients as it can be performed in an out-patient setting. The ultrasonographic appearance of local recurrence is identical to the primary tumour, i.e. echo-poor. It may, however, be difficult to differentiate between a recurrent tumour and fibrosis.[16] In such cases, needle biopsy guided by ERUS can provide the tissue diagnosis.[11] Female patients treated by restorative resection or abdominoperineal excision can also be scanned transvaginally.

The sonographic anatomy of the neorectum is no different from the original rectum apart from the fact that the anastmotic area may look more thickened than the rectal wall. Sometimes there may be a localised thickening in the wall due to the taenia of the colon that forms the neorectum following the surgery. The presence of staples does not usually affect the interpretation of the images as the staples are seen as small bright echoes. One must be wary about postoperative pelvic anatomy on ERUS because the uterus or a segment of small bowel may prolapse alongside the neo rectum and can be mistaken for recurrent tumour.

Endorectal ultrasonography may have a role in assessing extrarectal tumours such as leiomyosarcomas and rare forms of rectal malignancy such as carcinoids. Its role in evaluating such tumours is uncertain, as all series are small.

CONCLUSIONS

Endorectal ultrasonography is an objective and highly effective method of assessing rectal cancer pre-operatively, without exposing the patient to radiation. Interpretation of the ultrasonogram, owing to its dynamic nature, is highly operator-dependent. The biggest limitation of ERUS is the long learning curve. It requires a lot of experience to achieve expertise in this technique. The modern management of rectal cancer should include ERUS as it provides a basis for logical treatment planning. However, a review of the current literature suggests that there is little information about the impact of ERUS findings on clinical decision making. Critical evaluation of the real clinical value of ERUS is required and should involve comparison with other imaging techniques used in rectal cancer. Education, training and quality control in the use of ERUS also require further work.

In future, the development of smaller diameter probes with higher resolution transducers may reduce the current difficulties of examining the stenotic lesions and patients after radiotherapy. It should also lead to more accurate assessment of perirectal lymph nodes, especially lateral pelvic lymph nodes. Newer methods such as ERUS guided localised treatment of primary or recurrent tumours may bring new perspectives and expanded indications. The future relationship between MRI and ERUS is unresolved and may well be determined by the technical development of endoluminal MRI.

Acknowledgements

The authors would like to thank Professor B.J. Rowlands and Dr S.A. Watson for their support.

References

1. Swedish Rectal Cancer Trial. Improved survival with preoperative radiotherapy in resectable rectal cancer. N Engl J Med 1997; 336: 980–987
2. Dahlberg M, Glimelius B, Graf W, Pahlman L. Preoperative irradiation affects functional results after surgery for rectal cancer. Dis Colon Rectum 1998; 41: 543–551.
3. MacFarlane J K, Ryall R D H, Heald R J. Mesorectal excision for rectal cancer. Lancet 1993; 341: 457–460.
4. Banerjee A K, Jehle E C, Shorthouse A J. Local excision of rectal tumours. Br J Surg 1995; 82: 1165–1173.
5. Konishi F, Ugajin H, Ito K, Kanazawa K. Endorectal ultrasonography with a 7.5-MHz linear array scanner for the assessment invasion of rectal cancer. Int J Colorectal Dis 1990; 5: 15–20.
6. Wood C B, Gillis C R, Hole D, Malcolm A J H, Blumgart L H. Local tumour invasion as a prognostic factor in colorectal cancer. Br J Surg 1981; 68: 326–328.
7. Copeland E M, Miller L D, Jones R S. Prognostic factors in carcinoma of the colon and rectum. Am J Surg 1968; 116: 875–881.
8. Glaser F, Schlag P, Herfarth C. Endorectal ultrasonography for the assessment of invasion of rectal tumours and lymph node involvement. Br J Surg 1990; 77: 883–887.
9. Konishi F, Ugajin H, Ito K, Kanazawa K. Endorectal ultrasonography with a 7.5-MHz linear array scanner for the assessment of invasion of rectal cancer. Int J Colorect Dis 1990; 5: 15-20.
10. Katsura Y, Yamada K, Ishizawa T, Yoshinaka H, Shimazu H. Endorectal ultrasonography for the assessment of wall invasion and lymph node metastasis in rectal cancer. Dis Colon Rectum 1992; 35: 362–368.
11. Milsom J W, Czyrko C, Hull T L, Strong S A, Fazio V W. Pre-operative biopsy of pararectal lymph nodes in rectal cancer using endoluminal ultrasonography, Dis Colon Rectum 1994; 37: 364–368.
12. Tio T L, Coene P P, Van Delden O M, Tytgat G N. Colorectal carcinoma: pre-operative TNM classification with endosonography. Radiology 1991; 179: 165–170.
13. Tarroni D, Mascagni D, Urciuoli P, Di Pietrantonio M, Di Matteo. Endoluminal ultrasonographic accuracy in rectal cancer. Br J Surg 1992; 79: s30.
14. Thaler W, Watzka S, Martin F et al. Pre-operative staging of rectal cancer by endoluminal ultrasound vs magnetic resonance imaging. Dis Colon Rectum 1994; 37: 1189–1193.
15. Herzog U, Von Flue M, Tondelli P, Schuppiser J P. How accurate is endorectal ultrasound in the preoperative staging of rectal cancer? Dis Colon Rectum 1993; 36: 127–134.
16. Waizer A, Powsner E, Russo I et al. Prospective comparative study of magnetic resonance imaging versus transrectal ultrasound for preoperative staging and follow-up of rectal cancer: preliminary report. Dis Colon Rectum 1991; 34: 1068–1072.
17. Charnley R M, Pyf G, Amar S S, Hardcastle J D. The early detection of recurrent rectal carcinoma by rectal endosonography. Br J Surg 1988; 75: 1232.
18. Beynon J, Mortensen N J, Foy D M A. The detection and evaluation of locally recurrent rectal cancer with rectal endosonography. Dis Colon Rectum 1989; 32 : 509–517.
19. Solomon M J, McLeod R S. Endoluminal transrectal ultrasonography: accuracy, reliability and validity. Dis Colon Rectum 1993; 36: 200–205.
20. Sailer M, Leppert R, Bussen D, Fucks K H, Thiede A. Influence of tumour position on accuracy of endorectal ultrasound staging. Dis Colon Rectum 1997; 40: 1180-1186.
21. Akasu T, Sugihara K, Moriya Y, Fujita S. Limitations and pitfalls of transrectal ultrasonography for staging of rectal cancer. Dis Colon Rectum 1997; 40 (Suppl): s10–s15.
22. Beynon J, Mortensen N J, Rigby H, Channer J. Rectal endosonography accurately predicts depth of penetration in rectal cancer. Int J Colorect Dis 1992; 7: 4–7.
23. Yanagi H, Kusunoki M, Shoji Y, Yamamura T, Utsunomiya J. Pre-operative detection of distal intramural spread of lower rectal carcinoma using transrectal ultrasound. Dis Colon Rectum 1996; 39: 1210-1214.
24. Adams W J, Wong W D. Endorectal ultrasonic detection of malignancy within rectal villous lesions. Dis Colon Rectum 1995; 38: 1093–1096.
25. Napolean B, Pujol B, Berger F, Valette P J, Gerad J P, Souquet J C. Accuracy of endosonography in the staging of rectal cancer treated by radiotherapy. Br J Surg 1991; 78: 785–788.

26. Morija Y, Hojo K, Sawada T, Koyama Y. Significance of lateral node dissection for advanced rectal carcinoma at or below the peritoneal reflection. Dis Colon Rectum 1989; 32: 307–315.

27. Adams I J, Mohamdee M O, Martin IK G et al. Role of circumferential margin in the local recurrence of rectal cancer. Lancet 1994; 344: 707–711.

28. Hulsmans F-jh, Bosma A, Mulder P J J, Reeders J W A J, Tytgat G N J. Perirectal lymph nodes in rectal cancer: In vitro correlation of sonographic parameters and histological findings. Radiology 1992; 184: 533–560.

29. Rifkin M D, Ehrlich S M, Marks G. Staging of rectal carcinoma: prospective comparison of endorectal US and CT. Radiology 1989; 170: 319–322.

30. Milsom J W, Lavery I C, Stolfi V M et al. The expanding utility of endoluminal ultrasonography in the management of rectal cancer. Surgery 1992; 112: 832–841.

31. Lindmark G, Elvin A, Pahlman L, Glimelius B. The value of endosonography in pre-operative staging of rectal cancer. Int J Colorect Dis 1992; 7: 162–166.

32. Akasu T, Sunouchi K, Sawada T, Tsioulias G J, Muto T, Morioko Y. Preoperative staging of rectal carcinoma: prospective comparison of transrectal ultrasonography and computed tomography [abstract]. Gastroenterology 1990; 98: A268.

33. Van den Brekel M W M, Stel H V, Castelijins J A. Cervical lymph node assessment of radiologic criteria, Radiology 1990; 177: 379–384.

34. Reasbeck P G, Manktelow A, McArthur A M, Packer S G K, Berkeley B B. An evaluation of pelvic lymphoscintigraphy in the staging of colorectal carcinoma. Br J Surg 1984; 71: 936–940.

35. Stocchi L, Nelson H. Diagnostic and therapeutic applications of monoclonal antibodies in colorectal cancer. Dis Colon Rectum 1998; 41 : 232–250.

36. Abulafi A M, Williams S N. Local recurrence of rectal cancer; the problem, mechanism, management and adjuvant therapy. Br J Surg 1994; 81: 7–9.

37. Beynon J, Mortensen N J, Foy D M A, Channer J L, Rigby H, Virjee J. Pre-operative assessment of mesorectal lymph node involvement in rectal cancer. Br J Surg 1989; 76: 276–279.

38. Beynon J. An evaluation of the role of rectal endosonography in rectal cancer, Ann R Coll Surg Engl 1989; 71: 131–139.

39. Hildebrandt U, Beynon J, Feifel G, Mortensen N J. Endorectal sonography. In: Feifel G, Hildebrandt U, Mortensen N J (eds) Endosonography in Gastroenterology, Gynaecology and Urology. Berlin: Spring, 1990; 81–130.

40. Hildebrandt U, Klein G, Schwarz H P. Endosonography of pararectal lymph nodes. In vitro and in vivo evaluation. Dis Colon Rectum 1990; 33: 863–868.

S. J. Parker   P. E. Watkins

Immunomodulatory therapies of sepsis and SIRS

Inflammation is the body's non-specific response to cellular injury; the end result of highly amplified, yet tightly controlled, humoral and cellular mechanisms aimed principally at limiting tissue damage. Localised inflammation is an appropriate protective physiological response often eliminating the initiating noxious stimulus and restoring homeostasis. Loss of local control or an exaggerated host reaction can, however, result in a progressive illness, the systemic inflammatory response syndrome (SIRS), that, in extreme cases, can lead to organ dysfunction and death. SIRS can result from many aetiological triggers (e.g. burns, infection, pancreatitis, trauma) with sepsis defined as SIRS arising as a result of infection.[1] Despite advances in critical care medicine, the mortality associated with severe sepsis and septic shock has changed little over the past 20 years.[2] As sepsis is the commonest cause of death on adult intensive care units, new therapeutic approaches, effective irrespective of the infecting organism, need to be identified.

In this chapter, the general properties of the mediators that control the immuno-inflammatory cascade will be outlined. This will be followed by a discussion of those immunomodulatory therapies, used as an adjunct to organ support, that have shown the most promising results in human randomised

---

- As sepsis is the commonest cause of death on adult intensive care units, new therapeutic approaches, effective irrespective of the infecting organism, need to be identified.

Surgeon Lieutenant Commander S. J. Parker BSc MS FRCS FRCS(Ed) Royal Navy, Surgical Specialist Registrar, Biomedical Sciences, Defence Evaluation and Research Agency, Porton Down, Salisbury SP4 0JQ, UK

Dr P. E. Watkins MA VetMB PhD MRCVS, Veterinary Officer, Biomedical Sciences, Defence Evaluation and Research Agency, Porton Down, Salisbury SP4 0JQ, UK

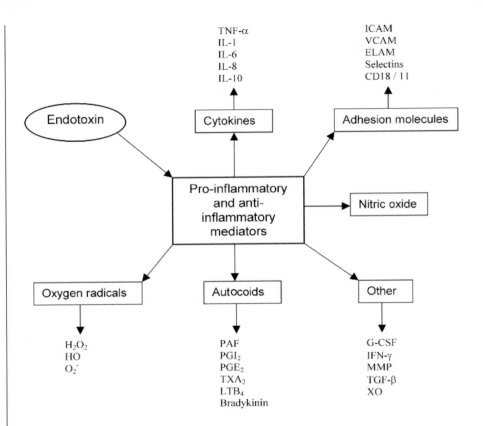

Fig. 1 Pro-inflammatory and anti-inflammatory mediators.

controlled trials (RCTs). The reasons for the apparent failure of many of these studies will be highlighted.

GENERAL PROPERTIES OF CYTOKINES

A co-ordinated immuno-inflammatory response requires the regulation of many cell types achieved principally by the actions of soluble protein (cytokine) and lipid or peptide (autocoid) mediators released by macrophages, neutrophils, lymphocytes, platelets and the endothelium (Fig. 1). Some cytokines, including tumour necrosis factor-alpha (TNFα), interleukin-1 (IL-1) and IL-8 have pro-inflammatory actions whilst others, such as IL-4, IL-10, IL-13, have predominantly counter-regulatory activities.[3] 'Proximal' cytokines, including TNFα and IL-1, are released early in the inflammatory process whilst 'distal' cytokines, for example IL-6 and IL-8, are released later in this pathological continuum.

Cytokines and autocoids regulate both the amplitude and duration of the inflammatory response, having multiple effects on cell differentiation and also considerable overlap and redundancy in their actions. The response induced by a particular mediator depends on its concentration, the cell type on which it is acting, the presence of other modulatory peptides and the availability of receptors. In an attempt to control and localise an inflammatory process both pro- and anti-inflammatory mediators are simultaneously released. The balance between these two competing mechanisms is vital if homeostasis is to be maintained. An exaggerated anti-inflammatory response can result in immunosuppression, whereas an excessive pro-inflammatory response can produce systemic overflow of cytokines.[4] The physiological responses induced by inflammatory mediators are invariably the result of their paracrine actions.[5] Their often compartmentalised production results in serum concentrations that do not accurately reflect local physiological levels.[6] Quite aptly, Cavaillon et al[7] have described serum cytokine concentrations as being the 'tip of the iceberg'.

Key point 1

- Both pro- and anti-inflammatory mediators are released following an initiating trigger and tightly control the immuno-inflammatory cascade. Derangement of either response can result in systemic sepsis or SIRS.

IMMUNOMODULATORY THERAPIES

The treatment of severe sepsis and septic shock has, until recently, centred around the eradication of established infection with surgery or antibiotics, accompanied by intensive organ support. With the realisation that the pathological effects of sepsis and SIRS can result both from the direct actions of micro-organisms and their toxins and indirectly from the host response, recent interest has been shown in novel immunomodulatory therapies (Fig. 2). These have attempted to attenuate the actions of bacterial toxins, to limit the host inflammatory response or to reduce tissue damage resulting from the established inflammatory process.[3] Anti-cytokine therapies have attempted to either inhibit pro-inflammatory or enhance anti-inflammatory responses. A delicate balance does, however, need to be achieved between the inhibition of an excessive response and ablation of essential host defences. Many strategies have been investigated in animal studies, a limited number have progressed to clinical trials, but disappointingly few have shown any significant therapeutic effect.

ENDOTOXIN

Endotoxin or lipopolysaccharide (LPS) is found within the external membrane of the cell wall of Gram-negative bacteria and is released from growing and damaged organisms. LPS binds to a number of different serum carrier molecules the most important of which is lipopolysaccharide binding protein (LBP). The LPS–LBP complex interacts with monocytes and macrophages mainly via the CD14 cell-surface receptor. LPS, and in particular its lipid A

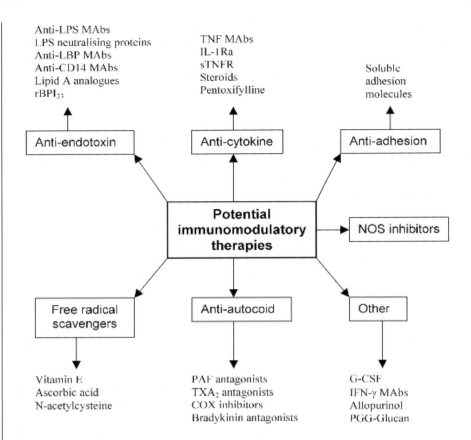

Anti-LPS MAbs
LPS neutralising proteins
Anti-LBP MAbs
Anti-CD14 MAbs
Lipid A analogues
rBPI$_{23}$

TNF MAbs
IL-1 Ra
sTNFR
Steroids
Pentoxifylline

Soluble
adhesion
molecules

Anti-endotoxin

Anti-cytokine

Anti-adhesion

**Potential
immunomodulatory
therapies**

NOS inhibitors

Free radical
scavengers

Anti-autocoid

Other

Vitamin E
Ascorbic acid
N-acetylcysteine

PAF antagonists
TXA$_2$ antagonists
COX inhibitors
Bradykinin antagonists

G-CSF
IFN-γ MAbs
Allopurinol
PGG-Glucan

Fig. 2 Potential immunomodulatory therapies.

component, is a potent stimulator of cytokine production. Administration of endotoxin to healthy human volunteers produces clinical features of sepsis[8] and elevated serum endotoxin levels have been demonstrated in some,[9] but not all,[10] studies of patients with severe sepsis.

Anti-endotoxin therapies

A number of approaches have been investigated as potential mechanisms for limiting the pathological effects of LPS. In early studies, polyclonal human antisera with high levels of anti-LPS antibodies were shown to reduce the mortality of Gram-negative sepsis[11] and to be effective as prophylaxis against Gram-negative infection in high risk surgical patients.[12] Following technological advances, anti-LPS monoclonal antibodies (MAbs) were developed of which HA-1A (Centoxin®) and E5 (Xoma®) have been the most extensively studied. HA-1A is a human anti-lipid A IgM antibody derived from the spleen of a patient vaccinated with the J5 rough mutant of *Escherichia coli*. E5 is a similar murine anti-lipid A IgM MAb. Each binds to different epitopes of the lipid A component of LPS.[13] Despite encouraging results from animal studies, RCTs of both of these agents have been disappointing. Three large trials of HA-1A, which enrolled over 3,000 patients with septic shock, failed to show any survival benefit.[14–16] A subgroup analysis of 200 patients with Gram-negative bacteraemia from the study of Ziegler et al[14] showed improved survival, but, the validity of such *post hoc* retrospective analyses has been questioned.[17,18] HA-1A was granted a product licence in Europe in 1992, but, was withdrawn from the market in 1993. Two large trials of E5, which recruited over 1,500 patients, similarly showed no reduction in mortality in patients with severe sepsis.[19,20] There was, however, an improvement with antibody treatment in the extent of organ dysfunction and mortality in those with proven Gram-negative infection in one of these studies.[19]

Other therapeutic approaches that have attempted to limit the pathological effects of LPS include anti-CD14 MAbs, anti-LBP MAbs, lipid A analogues and LPS neutralising proteins. Bactericidal/permeability increasing (BPI) protein is a 55–60 kDa neutrophil primary granule protein, structurally similar to LBP. It has a higher affinity for LPS than LBP and is able to remove LPS from the LPS–LBP complex. In healthy volunteer studies, a recombinant 23 kDa N-terminal fragment ($rBPI_{23}$) has been shown to abolish the cytokine response to an endotoxin challenge.[21] To date, no large-scale RCTs of these agents have been reported but a multinational placebo-controlled trial of $rBPI_{23}$ in meningococcal sepsis is currently in progress.[22]

Key point 2

- No anti-endotoxin therapy has been shown to produce a survival benefit in randomised, placebo-controlled trials of patients with severe sepsis and septic shock.

TUMOUR NECROSIS FACTOR-ALPHA

TNFα is a 17 kDa polypeptide produced predominantly by cells of the reticulo-endothelial system. It has a pivotal role in sepsis and SIRS with a short half-life; there is tight control of its expression at both the transcriptional, translational and post-translational processing levels. It acts directly on cells as well as stimulating the release of other inflammatory mediators. It also appears to be important in inducing apoptosis and attenuating inflammatory responses. In healthy human volunteers, a low-dose TNFα infusion produces clinical features of sepsis[23] and in some studies, elevated serum TNFα levels have been demonstrated in patients with severe sepsis.[24]

Anti-TNFα therapies

Anti-TNFα therapies, in particular the use of anti-TNFα MAbs, have been extensively investigated in both animal and clinical studies and have proved to be some of the more promising immunomodulatory treatments of sepsis and SIRS. Bay x1351 is an IgG_1 anti-TNFα MAb with a half-life of approximately 50 h.[25] It has been used as a single intravenous infusion in three large RCTs of patients with severe sepsis and septic shock of less than 12 h duration. The NORASEPT I trial randomised 971 patients (478 with septic shock) to receive 7.5 mg/kg, 15 mg/kg anti-TNFα MAb or placebo.[26] No improvement in 28-day mortality was identified. A subgroup analysis showed a significant reduction in mortality at 3 days in those patients with septic shock at study entry. The INTERSEPT trial randomised 563 patients (420 with septic shock) to receive 3 mg/kg, 15 mg/kg anti-TNFα MAb or placebo.[27] It also failed to show an improvement in 28-day mortality, but, more rapid shock reversal and a reduction in the extent of organ dysfunction was seen in the antibody-treated groups. As a result of the above studies, NORASEPT II recruited only patients with septic shock and reported in early 1998.[28] A total of 1879 patients received either 7.5 mg/kg anti-TNFα MAb or placebo. No difference in mortality or shock reversal was seen between the two treatment arms.

CB0006 is a murine anti-TNFα MAb that, in a study of 80 patients with severe sepsis or septic shock, also failed to show any survival benefit.[29] A subgroup analysis showed that, compared with historical controls, an improved outcome was seen in those with high plasma TNFα levels at study entry. MAK 195F is a 'humanised' $F(ab')_2$ fragment of a murine IgG directed against human TNFα. It too produced no survival benefit in a study of 120 patients with severe sepsis, but retrospective stratification by serum IL-6 concentration suggested beneficial effects in those with elevated levels of this cytokine at study entry.[30]

TNFα exerts its biological effects through two receptor subtypes with molecular weights of 55 kDa and 75 kDa, respectively. Each has distinct and separate functions and different affinities for TNFα. Soluble TNFα receptors (sTNFR) have been demonstrated in the serum of patients with sepsis in approximately a 10 times concentration excess relative to TNFα.[8] They compete with membrane-bound receptors for TNFα and appear to be important in regulating TNFα responses. The therapeutic use of sTNFRs in sepsis has been evaluated using chimeric dimers of either the 55 kDa or 75 kDa sTNFR attached to the Fc portion of a human IgG bioengineered to increase TNFα affinity and reduce the rate of degradation. A large trial of sTNFR75 produced disappointing results with a significantly increased mortality observed in the treatment group.[31] A trial of sTNFR55, that enrolled almost 500 patients with severe sepsis, showed a trend towards a reduction in 28-day mortality that became significant when predicted mortality and plasma IL-6 levels were included in a prospectively planned logistic regression analysis.[32]

Other pharmacological agents have been shown to attenuate TNFα responses. Corticosteroids inhibit TNFα translation, but, despite encouraging results from animal studies, clinical trials in septic patients failed to demonstrate a survival benefit and to be associated with an increase in secondary nosocomial infection.[33] Phosphodiesterase inhibitors, particularly pentoxifylline, inhibit TNFα gene transcription, thalidomide destabilises TNFα mRNA and matrix

---

Key point 3

- Despite reductions in morbidity, no anti-TNFα therapy has been shown to reduce mortality in placebo-controlled, randomised controlled trials of patients with severe sepsis and septic shock.

metalloproteinases inhibitors block post-translational processing of TNFα. None, to date, has been extensively investigated in large-scale RCTs.

THE INTERLEUKINS

The interleukins are a class of cytokines produced by many different cell types. IL-1 and IL-8 have pro-inflammatory actions, whilst IL-4 and IL-10 have predominantly anti-inflammatory actions. IL-6 is regarded by many as one of the best available serum markers of the severity of inflammation.[34] IL-1 is a key mediator in the immuno-inflammatory cascade, interacting closely with other cytokines, particularly TNFα. Infusion of IL-1 in healthy volunteers produces clinical features of sepsis.[35] Increased IL-1 levels have been recorded in patients with severe sepsis,[9] with levels often correlating with the severity of the inflammatory process.[36]

Anti-IL-1 therapies

The most extensively investigated therapy directed against IL-1 has been the IL-1 receptor antagonist (IL-1Ra). This naturally occurring protein binds to the IL-1 receptor without causing cellular activation. Since only a few IL-1 receptors need to be activated in order to produce a response, a large excess of IL-1Ra is needed in order to inhibit its actions. In clinical trials of IL-1Ra, initially encouraging results were obtained. A phase II study reported a dose-dependent reduction in APACHE II scores and improvement in 28-day mortality in 99 patients with severe sepsis.[37] However, two subsequent multi-centre placebo-controlled RCTs, that enrolled over 1,800 patients, failed to confirm these results.[38,39]

OTHER POTENTIAL IMMUNOMODULATORY THERAPIES

The autocoids are important mediators in the immuno-inflammatory cascade and include the arachidonic acid derivatives – prostacyclin (PGI_2), thromboxane A_2 (TXA_2), the prostaglandins (particularly PGE_2) and the leukotrienes (particularly LTB_4). Cyclo-oxygenase (COX) is an enzyme central to the production of these phospholipid derivatives and COX inhibitors appear to have some beneficial effects in septic patients. Following promising animal and pilot studies, a large multicentre randomised placebo-controlled trial of ibuprofen in the treatment of sepsis was performed.[40] It enrolled 455 patients, half of whom were given intravenous ibuprofen (10 mg/kg up to a maximum of 800 mg) every 6 h for 2 days. Ibuprofen reduced serum lactate and systemic oxygen consumption, but produced no survival advantage. Selective TXA_2 inhibition may be preferable to non-selective COX inhibition as PGI_2 synthesis would be maintained. The azole anti-fungal agent ketoconazole is a selective thromboxane synthetase inhibitor and in a small-placebo controlled trial of 400 mg ketoconazole administered daily to patients with severe sepsis, a significant reduction in 30-day mortality was observed.[41]

Platelet activating factor (PAF) is a potent lipid pro-inflammatory mediator produced by the endothelium, neutrophils and platelets. Increased serum levels have been demonstrated in patients with severe sepsis and treatment with the naturally occurring PAF antagonist, BN 52021, produced encouraging results in a phase II RCT of 262 patients with severe sepsis.[42] A retrospectively defined subgroup of 120 patients with Gram-negative infection, treated with the PAF antagonist, showed a significant reduction in mortality from 57% to 33%. No improvement was seen in those with Gram-positive sepsis or in those patients in whom no organisms were identified. A recently reported phase III study, which recruited over 600 patients, unfortunately failed to confirm these results.[43] A small study (28 patients) of the PAF antagonist TCV-309 showed improved pulmonary and haematological function but no reduction in mortality in patients with SIRS or sepsis.[44]

Bradykinin is a potent pro-inflammatory mediator that is a potent stimulator of the production of other autocoids and nitric oxide. The bradykinin antagonist, CP 0127, has been shown in two RCTs, that recruited over 750 patients, to produce no survival benefit in those with SIRS presumed to be due to infection.[45,46] A survival benefit was, however, apparent in a prospectively defined subgroup of patients with proven Gram-negative infection. Other potential immunomodulatory therapies include nitric oxide synthase inhibition, soluble adhesion molecules, free radical scavengers, colony-stimulating factors, and biological response modifiers (e.g. PGG-glucan). Many have shown some benefit in small-scale clinical studies but, none been has been investigated in large-scale RCTs.

Key point 4

- The role of anti-autocoid therapies, nitric oxide inhibition, soluble adhesion molecules, free radical scavengers, colony stimulating factors and biological response modifiers in sepsis has still to be identified.

WHY HAVE SEPSIS TRIALS FAILED?

Despite encouraging results from animal studies, no immunomodulatory therapy has to date been shown to confer unequivocal benefit in large-scale clinical RCTs. This is especially disappointing in view of the current knowledge of the roles of the inflammatory mediators that have been targeted in these studies and the relative success of some of these agents in patients with chronic inflammatory states (e.g. ulcerative colitis, rheumatoid arthritis).[47] There are several reasons that appear to account for these divergent results.

Sepsis is an evolving pathological process with the different mediators varying in their relative importance throughout the progression of the response. Therapies targeted against a particular cytokine may be most effective if given during a critical time period and may be of limited benefit, or even cause adverse effects, if given outside a 'therapeutic window'.[48] This is especially so for agents directed against the 'proximal' cytokines which, in animal studies, have produced the more encouraging results when given prophylactically or immediately following the septic challenge. Following blockade of a 'proximal' cytokine, 'distal' pro-inflammatory mediators may continue to propagate the inflammatory response if treatment is given too late. Furthermore, massive redundancy exists within the immuno-inflammatory cascade with mediators displaying many overlapping actions. This, along with the synergistic action of many mediators, suggests that blockade of a single cytokine may not produce a balanced inhibition of the inflammatory response. The complexities of the immuno-inflammatory cascade are such that identifying a 'magic bullet' to produce a balanced reduction of cytokine responses may prove impossible and combination therapies may be more appropriate.[49]

Most preclinical sepsis studies have been performed using crude animal models that do not mimic well the clinical situation seen in man. In these studies, potential therapeutic agents have often been tested in a limited range of animals whose inflammatory responses often differ from those seen in man. Concerns have been voiced regarding the rapidity with which agents progress from simple animal studies to human trials without their efficacy being confirmed in clinically relevant models.[50,51] Animal studies are usually performed on sex-matched, genetically similar and healthy animals, whereas patients included in sepsis trials are by their very nature heterogeneous. Innate resistance to infection differs between individuals and age, immune status and drug therapies can all alter immuno-inflammatory responses. In animal studies, acute physiological parameters or short-term survival are invariably used as end-points. In clinical trials, 28-day mortality has often used as the primary end-point. The relevance of this one factor in assessing the overall efficacy of an immunomodulatory agent has been questioned, particularly when significant improvements in other secondary end-points have been identified.

In healthy human volunteers given an endotoxin infusion, cytokine levels vary greatly.[23] Similarly, in septic patients with similar levels of physiological derangement, markedly different cytokine and antagonist levels have been recorded.[24] In some patients, drugs that augment rather than inhibit the immunoinflammatory cascade may be the most appropriate form of therapy. Identification of clinical or serological markers that allow stratification of patients into groups who may benefit from a particular form of immuno-modulatory therapy is required. There is already some evidence to support this approach as, in many of the anti-TNFα MAb trials, patients were identified, with either proven Gram-negative infection[45] or elevated serum cytokine levels at study entry,[30] who appeared to show a survival benefit, but this has not been consistently repeated.[28,32] A genomic polymorphism has been identified within the TNFα gene locus that has been shown to influence serum TNFα levels and subsequent survival in patients with severe sepsis.[52] Recognition of such markers may also allow identification of high risk patients. With the poor reliability of serum cytokine levels to predict local mediator synthesis, assessment of tissue cytokine expression may provide additional information on the likely response to therapy. This is particularly so considering the increasingly recognised importance of the paracrine actions of cytokines. Furthermore, intravenous infusion of drugs, as used in most studies, may not be the optimal route of drug administration as most drugs are sequestered in the plasma compartment. At present, new and novel therapeutic agents are being developed at a faster rate than the ability to select who will benefit from them.

The disappointing results of the clinical trials of anti-cytokine therapies have led several authors to question the rationale for this therapeutic approach. A recent meta-analysis of 21 trials of non-glucocorticoid anti-inflammatory therapies identified a small, but statistically significant, benefit from these agents and suggested that, at best, they accounted for a 10% reduction in mortality.[53] It was concluded that many trials of immunomodulatory agents had enrolled insufficient patients. In order to reach statistical significance, it was estimated that up to 7,000 patients would be needed in some studies and, therefore, it seems that definitive answers regarding the potential benefit of many of these agents may never be known.

Key point 5

- Trials of immunomodulatory agents have been based on crude, inappropriate animal models. Clinical trials have failed, as the study populations have been too small and heterogeneous and the drugs were often given too late.

CONCLUSIONS

The complexities of the immuno-inflammatory cascade are such that pharmacological intervention has proved difficult. Despite encouraging results from animal studies, no immunomodulatory therapy has been shown to produce an unequivocal reduction in mortality in large-scale clinical sepsis trials. With the redundancy within the inflammatory cascade, it is unlikely that a single agent will produce a balanced inhibition and the use of combination therapies may prove more successful. In high risk patients, the prophylactic or early therapeutic use of immune stimulants followed by the later use of immunosuppressive agents may prove to be the most useful approach. The therapeutic benefit to be obtained from immunomodulatory agents is small and is unlikely to be realised in the absence of optimal resuscitation, surgery, antibiotics and intensive care therapy.

Key points for clinical practice

- Both pro- and anti-inflammatory mediators are released following an initiating trigger and tightly control the immuno-inflammatory cascade. Derangement of either response can result in systemic sepsis or SIRS.

- No anti-endotoxin therapy has been shown to produce a survival benefit in randomised, placebo-controlled trials of patients with severe sepsis and septic shock.

> ### *Key points for clinical practice (continued)*
>
> - Despite reductions in morbidity, no anti-TNFα therapy has been shown to reduce mortality in placebo-controlled, randomised controlled trials of patients with severe sepsis and septic shock.
>
> - The role of anti-autocoid therapies, nitric oxide inhibition, soluble adhesion molecules, free radical scavengers, colony stimulating factors and biological response modifiers in sepsis has still to be identified.
>
> - Trials of immunomodulatory agents have been based on crude, inappropriate animal models. Clinical trials have failed, as the study populations have been too small and heterogeneous and the drugs were often given too late.

References

1. Bone R C, Balk R A, Cerra F B et al and the ACCP/SCCM Consensus Conference Committee. American College of Chest Physicians/Society of Critical Care Medicine. Definitions of sepsis and organ failure and guidelines for the use of innovative therapies in sepsis. Chest 1992; 101: 1644–1655.
2. Sands K E, Bates D W, Lanken P N et al for the Academic Medical Centre Consortium Sepsis Project Working Group. Epidemiology of sepsis syndrome in 8 academic medical centres. JAMA 1997; 278: 234–240.
3. Lynn W A, Cohen J. Adjunctive therapy for septic shock: a review of experimental approaches. Clin Infect Dis 1995; 20: 143–158.
4. Bone R C. Towards a theory regarding the pathogenesis of the systemic inflammatory response syndrome: what we do and do not know about cytokine regulation. Crit Care Med 1996; 24: 163–172.
5. Schein M, Wittmann D H, Holzheimer R, Condon R E. Hypothesis: compartment-alization of cytokines in intra-abdominal infection. Surgery 1996; 119: 694–700.
6. Andrejko K M, Deutschman C S. Acute-phase gene expression correlates with intrahepatic tumor necrosis factor-α abundance but not with plasma tumor necrosis factor concentrations during sepsis/systemic inflammatory response syndrome in rats. Crit Care Med 1996; 24: 1947–1952.
7. Cavaillon J M, Munoz C, Fitting C, Misset B, Carlet J. Circulating cytokines: the tip of the iceberg. Circ Shock 1992; 38: 145–152.
8. Kuhns D B, Alvord W G, Gallin J. Increased circulating cytokines, cytokine antagonists and E-selectin after intravenous administration of endotoxin in humans. J Infect Dis 1995; 171: 145–152.
9. Casey L C, Balk R A, Bone R C. Plasma cytokine and endotoxin levels correlate with survival in patients with the sepsis syndrome. Ann Intern Med 1993; 119: 771–778.
10. Dofferhoff A S M, Bom V J J, De Vries-Hospers H G et al. Patterns of cytokines, plasma endotoxin, plasminogen activator inhibitor and acute phase proteins during the treatment of severe sepsis in humans. Crit Care Med 1992; 20: 185–192.
11. Ziegler E J, McCutchan J A, Fierer J et al. Treatment of Gram-negative bacteraemia and shock with human anti-serum to a mutant *Escherichia coli*. N Engl J Med 1982; 307: 1225–1230.
12. Baumgartner J-D, Glauser M P, McCutchan J A et al. Prevention of Gram-negative shock and death in surgical patients by antibody to endotoxin core glycolipid. Lancet 1985; ii: 59–63.
13. Fujihara Y, Bogard W C, Lei M-G, Daddona P E, Morrison D C. Monoclonal anti-lipid A IgM antibodies HA-1A and E5 recognise distinct epitopes on lipopolysaccharide and lipid A. J Infect Dis 1993; 168: 1429–1435.

14. Ziegler E J, Fisher C J, Sprung C L et al. Treatment of Gram-negative bacteremia and septic shock with HA-1A human monoclonal antibody against endotoxin. N Engl J Med 1991; 324: 429–436.

15. French National Registry of HA-1A. The French National Registry of HA-1A (Centoxin) in septic shock. A cohort study of 600 patients. The National Committee for the evaluation of Centoxin. Arch Intern Med 1994; 154: 2484–2491.

16. McCloskey R V, Straube R C, Sanders C, Smith S M, Smith C R for the CHESS Trial Study Group. Treatment of septic shock with human monoclonal antibody HA-1A. A randomised double-blind, placebo-controlled trial. Ann Intern Med 1994; 121: 1–5.

17. Dellinger R P. Post hoc analyses in sepsis trials: a formula for disappointment? Crit Care Med 1996; 24: 727–729.

18. Natanson C, Esposito C J, Banks S M. The sirens' songs of confirmatory sepsis trials: Selection bias and sampling error. Crit Care Med 1998; 26: 1927–1931.

19. Greenman R L, Schein R M H, Martin M A et al. A controlled trial of E5 murine monoclonal IgM antibody to endotoxin in the treatment of Gram-negative sepsis. JAMA 1991; 266: 1097–1102.

20. Bone R C, Balk R A, Fein A M et al and the E5 Sepsis Study Group. A second large controlled clinical study of E5, a monoclonal antibody to endotoxin: results of a prospective, multicenter, randomised controlled trial. Crit Care Med 1995; 23: 994–1005.

21. Von der Möhlen M A M, Kimmings A M, Wedel N I et al. Inhibition of endotoxin-induced cytokine release and neutrophil activation in humans by the use of recombinant bactericidal/permeability-increasing protein. J Infect Dis 1995; 172: 144–151.

22. Lynn W A. Anti-endotoxin therapeutic options for the treatment of sepsis. J Antimicrob Chemother 1998; 41 (Suppl A). 71–80.

23. Michie H R, Manogue K R, Spriggs D R et al. Detection of circulating tumour necrosis factor after endotoxin administration. N Engl J Med 1988; 318: 1481–1486.

24. Damas P, Canivet J-L, de Groote D et al. Sepsis and serum cytokine concentrations. Crit Care Med 1997; 25: 405–412.

25. Saravolatz L D, Wherry J C, Spooner C et al. Clinical safety, tolerability and pharmacokinetics of murine monoclonal antibody to human tumour necrosis factor-α. J Infect Dis 1994; 169: 214–217.

26. Abraham E, Wunderink R, Silverman H et al and the TNF-α MAb Sepsis Study Group. Efficacy and safety of monoclonal antibody to human tumor necrosis factor α in patients with sepsis syndrome. A randomised, controlled, double-blind, multicenter trial. JAMA 1995; 273: 934–941.

27. Cohen J, Carlet J and the INTERSEPT Study Group. INTERSEPT: an international multicenter placebo-controlled trial of monoclonal antibody to human TNF-α in patients with sepsis syndrome. Crit Care Med 1996; 24: 1431–1439.

28. Abraham E, Anzueto A, Gutierrez G et al and the NORASEPT II Study Group. Double-blind randomised controlled trial of monoclonal antibody to human tumour necrosis factor in treatment of septic shock. Lancet 1998; 351: 929–933.

29. Fisher C J, Opal S M, Dhainaut J-F et al. Influence of anti-tumor necrosis factor antibody on cytokine levels in patients with sepsis. Crit Care Med 1993; 21: 318–327.

30. Reinhart K, Wiegand-Löhnert C, Grimminger F et al. Assessment of the safety and efficacy of the monoclonal anti-tumour necrosis factor antibody fragment, MAK 195F, in patients with sepsis and septic shock: a multicentre, randomised, placebo-controlled, dose-ranging study. Crit Care Med 1996; 24: 733–742.

31. Fisher C J, Agosti J M, Opal S M et al. Treatment of septic shock with the tumor necrosis factor receptor:Fc fusion protein. N Engl J Med 1996; 334: 1697–1702.

32. Abraham E, Glauser M P, Butler T et al for the Ro 45-2081 Study Group. p55 tumor necrosis factor receptor fusion protein in the treatment of patients with severe sepsis and septic shock. JAMA 1997; 277: 1531–1538.

33. Lefering R, Neugebauer E A M. Steroid controversy in sepsis and septic shock. Crit Care Med 1995; 23: 1294–1303.

34. Damas P, Ledoux D, Nys M et al. Cytokine serum level during severe sepsis in human. IL-6 as a marker of severity. Ann Surg 1991; 215: 356–362.

35. Dinarello C A. Interleukin-1 and interleukin-1 antagonism. Blood 1991; 77: 1627–1652.

36. Waage A, Brandtzaeg P, Halstensen A, Kierulf P, Espevik T. The complex pattern of cytokines in serum from patients with meningococcal septic shock. Association between interleukin 6, interleukin 1 and fatal outcome. J Exp Med 1989; 69: 333–338.

37. Fisher C J, Slotman G J, Opal S M et al. Initial evaluation of human recombinant interleukin-1 receptor antagonist in the treatment of sepsis syndrome: a randomised. open-label, placebo-controlled multicentre trial. Crit Care Med 1994; 22: 12–21.

38. Fisher C J, Dhainaut J-F, Opal S M et al for the Phase III rhIL-1Ra Sepsis Syndrome Study Group. Recombinant interleukin-1 receptor antagonist in the treatment of patients with sepsis syndrome: results from a randomised double-blind placebo controlled trial. JAMA 1994; 271: 1836–1843.

39. Opal S M, Fisher C J, Dhainaut J-F A et al. Confirmatory interleukin-1 receptor antagonist trial in severe sepsis. A phase III, randomised, double-blind, placebo-controlled, multicentre trial. Crit Care Med 1997; 25: 1115–1124.

40. Bernard G R, Wheeler A P, Russell J A et al. The effects of ibuprofen on the physiology and survival of patients with sepsis. N Engl J Med 1997; 336: 912–918.

41. Yu M, Tomasa G. A double-blind, prospective, randomised trial of ketoconazole, a thromboxane synthetase inhibitor, in the prophylaxis of the adult respiratory distress syndrome. Crit Care Med 1993; 21: 1635–1642.

42. Dhainaut J-F A, Tenaillon A, Le-Tulzo et al. Platelet-activating factor receptor antagonist BN 52021 in the treatment of severe sepsis: a randomised, double-blind placebo controlled, multicentre clinical trial. Crit Care Med 1994; 22: 1720–1728.

43. Dhainaut J-F, Tenaillon A, Hemmer M et al for the BN 52021 Sepsis Investigator Group. Confirmatory platelet-activating factor receptor antagonist trial in patients with severe Gram-negative bacterial sepsis: a phase III, randomised, double-blind, placebo-controlled, multicentre trial. Crit Care Med 1998, 26: 1963–1971.

44. Froon A M F, Greve J W N, Buurman W A et al. Treatment with the platelet-activating factor antagonist TCV-309 in patients with severe systemic inflammatory response syndrome: a prospective, multicentre, double-blind, randomised phase II trial. Shock 1996; 5: 313–319.

45. Fein A M, Bernard G R, Criner G J et al for the CP 0127 SIRS and Sepsis Study Group. Treatment of severe systemic inflammatory response syndrome and sepsis with a novel bradykinin antagonist, Deltibant (CP 0127). JAMA 1997; 277: 482–487.

46. Rodell T C, Foster C. Sepsis data show negative trend in second phase II sepsis trial. Press release. Denver, Cortech, July 18 1995.

47. Moreland L W, Baumgartner S W, Schiff M H et al. Treatment of rheumatoid arthritis with a recombinant human tumor necrosis factor receptor (p75)-Fc fusion protein. N Engl J Med 1997; 337: 141–147.

48. Ridings P C, Windsor A C J, Sugerman H J et al. Beneficial cardiopulmonary effects of pentoxifylline in experimental sepsis are lost once septic shock is established. Arch Surg 1994; 130: 1199–1208.

49. Vincent J-L. Search for effective immunomodulating strategies against sepsis. Lancet 1998; 351: 922–923.

50. Piper R D, Cook D J, Bone R C, Sibbald W J. Introducing critical appraisal to studies of animal models investigating novel therapies in sepsis. Crit Care Med 1996; 24: 2059–2070.

51. Deitch E A. Animal models of sepsis and shock: a review and lessons learned. Shock 1998; 9: 1–11.

52. Stüber F, Petersen M, Bokelmann F et al. A genomic polymorphism within the tumour necrosis factor locus influences plasma tumour necrosis factor-alpha concentrations and outcome of patients with severe sepsis. Crit Care Med 1996; 24: 381–384.

53. Zeni F, Freeman B, Natanson C. Anti-inflammatory therapies to treat sepsis and septic shock: a reassessment. Crit Care Med 1997; 25: 1095–1100.

Edward R. Howard

Hepatobiliary surgery in children

THE BILE DUCTS

The biliary tract can be affected by a variety of disorders in infancy and childhood. The abnormalities may be congenital or acquired in origin, and may present with a wide range of symptoms and signs which include jaundice, pancreatitis, peritonitis or an abdominal mass. Recent developments in antenatal ultrasonography have allowed the detection of some congenital abnormalities of the biliary tract *in utero*.

The most frequent abnormality is biliary atresia. This is the end result of an inflammatory destruction of the bile ducts and has an incidence of approximately one per 14,000 live births. This condition usually presents with jaundice within the first 3–4 weeks of life. Inspissation of viscid bile and spontaneous perforation of the common bile duct also occur in early infancy and may be mistaken for atresia.

Congenital cystic dilatations of the biliary tract may present at any age but the majority are diagnosed before 10 years.

Gallstones are most commonly associated with haemolytic disorders, particularly in patients with sickle cell disease, but cholesterol cholelithiasis may also occur in young children.

BILIARY ATRESIA

The inflammatory lesion which results in obliteration of the lumen of the extrahepatic bile ducts is also associated with intrahepatic pathology which has been likened to sclerosing cholangitis. Intrahepatic histological changes include widening of the portal tracts with oedema and fibrosis, bile stasis and proliferation of bile ductules. The extent of the occlusion of the extrahepatic

---

Professor Edward R. Howard MS FRCS FRCSE, 5 High Standing, Chaldon Common Road, Chaldon, Surrey CR3 5DY, UK

ducts varies from case to case but the commonest finding at operation is of an occlusion up to the capsule of the liver in the porta hepatis. Early descriptions of cases of biliary atresia divided them into 'correctable' or 'non-correctable' depending on the presence or absence of a residual segment of patent duct at the upper end of the biliary tract. However, the development of the operation of porto-enterostomy, which is frequently followed by satisfactory biliary drainage after excision of a totally occluded biliary tract, has led to the acceptance of a classification devised by the Japanese Society of Pediatric Surgeons[1] (Fig. 1) which describes three main types:

Type 1 – *atresia of the common bile duct and a patent segment of hepatic duct which may be in communication with the gallbladder.*

Type 2 – *atresia of the common hepatic duct with patency of segments of the right and left hepatic ducts.*

Type 3 – *atresia of the right and left hepatic ducts which are replaced with a mass of chronic inflammatory tissue containing biliary ductules which communicate with residual intrahepatic ducts.[2] The size of the inflammatory mass in the porta hepatis varies in size from case to case and tends to diminish with the child's age.[2]*

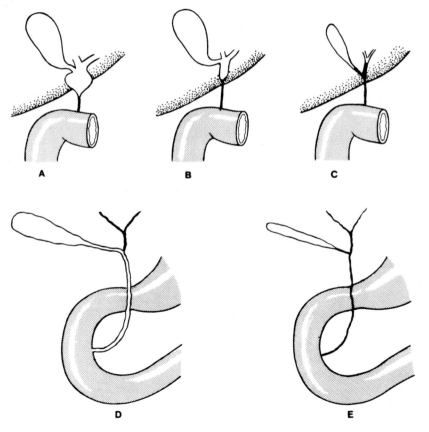

Fig. 1 Diagrammatic representation of some of the variations in bile duct occlusion observed in biliary atresia. A and B are examples of type 1, C of type 2, and D and E of type 3 in the Japanese classification.

Type 1 and type 2 cases are unusual and account for only 12% of the total. The majority (88%) are of the type 3 variety.

The aetiology of biliary atresia remains unknown, although an embryological event at around the 11th week of gestation is suggested by the association with other extrahepatic abnormalities, such as the biliary atresia-splenic malformation syndrome (BASM)[3] in which abnormalities of the spleen (usually polysplenia but occasionally asplenia) and portal vein accompany the bile duct lesions. This timing is supported by an absence of the liver enzyme γ-glutamyl transpeptidase (GGT) in amniotic fluid samples taken from fetuses with biliary atresia. This enzyme is normally found in the amniotic fluid from the 2nd trimester onwards and relates to *in utero* bile production and defaecation.[4] Biliary atresia has also been detected on antenatal ultrasonography in three cases.[5]

Maternal or perinatal inoculation of animals with hepatotropic viruses, such as reovirus or rotavirus, can result in some of the features of biliary atresia,[6,7] although viral studies in affected patients have proved negative.

Embryological studies of the complex development of the biliary tract have shown interesting similarities between the histology of the porta hepatis in patients who have undergone surgery and the developing human biliary tract examined between 11–13 weeks gestation. It has been suggested, from these observations, that biliary atresia may be the result of an arrested development of biliary radicles.[8]

Treatment

It is now generally accepted that the operation known as porto-enterostomy[9] is the primary treatment for infants with biliary atresia and that liver transplantation should be reserved for those who do not achieve satisfactory bile drainage or for those who develop the complications of progressive liver failure. The initial step in the operation is a complete mobilisation of the liver which is rotated to expose the porta hepatis. The exposure of the porta hepatis is excellent in the young infant. The atretic biliary tract is excised completely from the supraduodenal border to the capsule of the liver above the bifurcation of the portal vein which is mobilised downwards. Biliary continuity is achieved by anastomosing a Roux-en-Y loop of jejunum to the edges of the transected porta hepatis. The crucial part of the operation is the accurate dissection and excision of the inflammatory tissue in the porta hepatis out as far as the origin of the right and left hepatic ducts.[9]

The achievement of satisfactory volumes of bile drainage is related to the age of the infant at surgery,[10] and the size of the residual bile ductules at the porta hepatis.[11] Poor surgical results have also been associated with a small number of ductules in the porta hepatis and to an absence of significant portal inflammatory changes.

Long-term results

An analysis of long-term outcome in 184 cases treated by one surgeon between 1980–1989 showed the relationship of age at the time of surgery. The success rate of porto-enterostomy performed before 8 weeks of age was 67% compared with 36% for those treated later.[12] The overall 5-year survival rate was approximately 39% and collected figures from the major long-term series showed similar results for survival at 5 and 10 years after porto-enterostomy.[13]

Key point 1
- Early surgery is essential in biliary atresia.

Analysis of the collected series showed that, although survival was similar at 5 and 10 years, the number who remained free from jaundice diminished from 25% to 16%.

Postoperative progress in these patients may be complicated by cholangio-hepatitis, progressive hepatic fibrosis and portal hypertension, and, occasionally, by hepatopulmonary syndrome or pulmonary hypertension.[14] Hepatopulmonary syndrome is recognised by hypoxia and cyanosis which worsens on standing or exercise and which is secondary to intrapulmonary shunting and vascular dilatation. The aetiology may be related to vasoactive substances, such as endothelin and prostaglandin F_2, which are either not metabolised by the liver or which are secreted by endothelial cells.

Of 22 patients in one series who have survived for more than 20 years after porto-enterostomy,[15] 16 have near normal lives; successful pregnancies have been recorded by other authors.[13] A significant proportion of patients will require liver transplantation either because of a failure to establish bile flow after porto-enterostomy or because of progressive liver disease in spite of remission of jaundice. The early results of transplantation are encouraging and Goss et al,[16] for example, reported 1, 2 and 5-year actuarial survival rates of 83%, 80% and 78%, respectively. Approximately 16% of the patients underwent repeat liver grafting on more than one occasion.

Key point 2
- Porto-enterostomy for biliary atresia can result in good bile flow and long-term survival has been proven.

In summary, there has been a remarkable change in outcome for children with biliary atresia in the last 30 years. The only long-term survivors before this time were rare cases of type 1 disease who had undergone a successful biliary-enteric anastomosis via a residual patent segment of bile duct. Treatment with either porto-enterostomy or hepatic transplantation can now result in long-term survival in more than 90% of cases.

CHOLEDOCHAL CYST

Congenital cystic dilatation of the biliary tract is a rare abnormality which may be complicated by jaundice, cholangitis, gall stones and carcinoma. The true incidence is unknown, although in one study it accounted for 1 case in 26,000 admissions in a London hospital.[17] More than 60% are diagnosed in children under 10 years of age and there is a female:male ratio of 4:1 in all large series. The accepted classification (Fig. 2) recognises 5 types of cystic dilatation:[18]

Type 1c – extrahepatic cystic dilatation.

Type 1f – extrahepatic fusiform dilatation.

Type 2 – diverticulum of the common bile duct.

Type 3 – choledochocele.

Type 4 – combined intra- and extrahepatic cysts.

Type 5 – intrahepatic cysts.

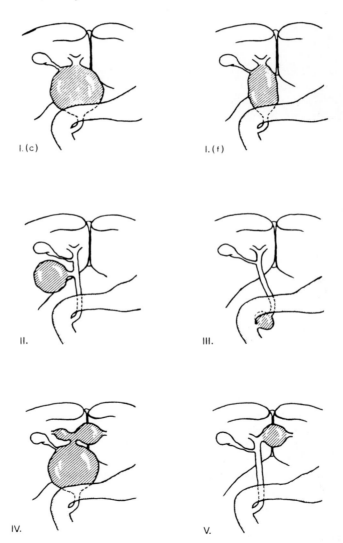

Fig. 2 Diagrammatic representation of the standard classification of choledochal cysts (after Todani et al[18]).

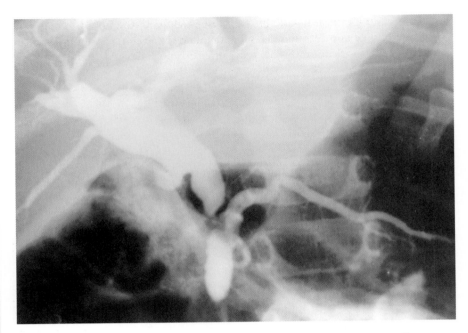

Fig. 3 ERCP of a fusiform choledochal cyst showing a long common pancreatico-biliary channel. The 7-year-old child presented with a history of pancreatitis.

Types 2 an 3 are rare and were not identified in a series of 78 children, 56% of whom presented with type 1c cysts. Fusiform dilatation (type 1f) occurred in 36%, and the rarer type 4 and type 5 lesions in only 8%.[19]

The classic presentation of a triad of jaundice, pain and a mass in the right hypochondrium is rare and was found in only 4 (6%) of 78 children.[19] The most frequent presentations were jaundice (69%), and pain (18%).

The antenatal diagnosis of choledochal cysts in 10 cases at a mean gestational age of 20 weeks emphasises the embryological origin of the condition[20] and offers the possibility of early definitive surgery. However, most cases are only diagnosed after the onset of obstructive jaundice, which may be intermittent, or of pancreatitis. Pancreatitis is associated with a common pancreatico-biliary channel (Fig. 3) in which the pancreatico-biliary junction lies outside the duodenal wall, allowing free reflux of pancreatic enzymes into the biliary tract.[21,22] This anatomical feature was identified in 42 (76%) of 55 symptomatic choledochal cysts.[19]

Key point 3

- Jaundice and/or pancreatitis are frequent presentations of choledochal cysts.

Pathology

Komi et al[23] have devised a complete classification of pancreatico-biliary channels based on the radiographic appearances of 51 cases and they suggested that chronic pancreatitis is associated with certain sub-types even after appropriate surgery for the cystic abnormality of the bile duct. There are 2 main types of pancreatico-biliary union; either the bile duct appears to join the pancreatic duct or the pancreatic duct appears to join the bile duct. These variations may be important in determining complications and Misra and Dwivedi[24] noted that the angle of insertion of the bile duct into the pancreatic duct was greater in those patients with a history of pancreatitis (mean angle of 40°) than in those without (mean angle of 21°).

The term 'forme fruste' choledochal cyst has been used to describe an association of long common channel with pathological changes in the wall of the bile ducts typical of choledochal cyst, but without significant dilatation of the bile ducts.[25] The patients may present with cholangitis, pancreatitis or bile duct calculi; the treatment is duct excision and Roux-en-Y bile duct drainage.

Key point 4

- Pancreatitis in childhood may be associated with a common pancreatico-biliary channel.

Histologically, choledochal cyst walls show chronic inflammatory change and partial loss of epithelium. These features have been related to age and in a study of 40 cases there were typical changes of epithelial loss and fibrosis under 2 years of age with increasing inflammatory features in older patients. By 15 years, there was severe epithelial loss and young adults showed metaplastic changes. Adenocarcinoma was identified in 5 of the 23 excised cysts.[26] High levels of phospholipid A_2 have been identified in bile from patients with common channels and it has been suggested that the production of a cytotoxic phospholipid might be the cause of the mucosal damage.[27]

Anomalous pancreatico-biliary junctions have now been associated with the development of gall bladder carcinoma in adults. A series of 18 patients with anomalous junctions without choledochal cysts were analyzed retrospectively[28] and, in 16 patients, there were gall bladder abnormalities including carcinoma ($n = 8$), and mucosal hyperplasia ($n = 11$).

Spontaneous rupture and biliary peritonitis is a rare, but well documented, complication of choledochal cysts.[19,29] In a recent review, perforation was documented in 13 out of 187 cases[30] and all of the patients were less than 4 years of age.

Treatment

Ultrasonography together with endoscopic or percutaneous cholangiography provide accurate methods of defining the anatomy of choledochal cysts and their associated pancreatico-biliary channels. Complete cyst excision of the extrahepatic lesions and Roux-en-Y reconstruction of the biliary tract is now the recommended treatment for choledochal cysts as the lesser operation of cyst-enterostomy is complicated by cholangitis, stone formation and anastomotic stenosis in approximately 40% of cases. Tan and Howard,[31] for example, reported good long-term results in 25 patients who underwent total cyst excision. In comparison, 5 of 9 patients who underwent a cystenterostomy in the same series suffered recurrent pancreatitis or cholangitis and needed subsequent re-operation and cyst excision.

Treatment of intrahepatic biliary cysts can be difficult. Drainage of bilateral cysts is improved by resection of any associated extrahepatic cysts and the construction of a wide Roux-en-Y anastomosis to the hepatic ducts. Unilateral cysts can be removed by partial hepatectomy if symptomatic.[32]

Key point 5

- Total excision is the treatment of choice for choledochal cysts.

INSPISSATED BILE

Infants may present in the neonatal period with obstructive jaundice secondary to impaction of thick bile or biliary 'sludge' in the lower portion of the common bile duct. In the past, this was commonly associated with excessive haemolysis secondary to rhesus or ABO blood group incompatibility. The development of early exchange transfusion for these conditions led to a reduction in the incidence of inspissated bile syndrome. Other aetiological factors include bowel dysfunction, dehydration, diuretic therapy, and cystic fibrosis. Parenteral nutrition has been a particular problem,[33] although it is not clear whether the viscid bile is a result of the parenteral nutrition or to failure of gut activity. The use of cholecystokinin to stimulate gall bladder activity and increase bile flow has been suggested as a prophylactic measure.

Many of the infants have other problems such as prematurity, respiratory distress syndrome and intra-abdominal sepsis.[34]

The clinical presentation of inspissated bile syndrome may be mistaken for biliary atresia, but ultrasonography of the biliary tract reveals a dilated system and the inspissated material may be seen in the lower bile duct. The diagnosis can be confirmed with percutaneous cholangiography, which may also be used to flush the bile duct clear. Occasionally, operative exploration of the bile duct is necessary to relieve the obstruction.

SPONTANEOUS PERFORATION OF THE BILE DUCT

Acute perforation of the bile duct occurs typically at between 2–6 weeks of age. The perforation is always found at the junction of the cystic duct and the common bile duct which supports the suggestion of an area of developmental weakness.[35] Obstruction with inspissated bile has been demonstrated in several of the affected infants[36] and is a likely cause of high intraluminal pressure.

The infants usually have an uncomplicated birth history and develop normally until the onset of jaundice, pale stools and dark urine. Peritonitis is rare, but there is increasing abdominal distension from biliary ascites which may cause a diagnostic yellow staining of the inguinal and peri-umbilical regions. Biliary radionuclide scanning will confirm the leakage of bile into the general peritoneal cavity and operative cholangiography via the gallbladder will demonstrate the site of the perforation (Fig. 4). A small perforation may be sutured after confirming satisfactory flow of contrast into the duodenum, and temporary drainage is established via a cholecystostomy catheter. A large perforation may require T-tube drainage for approximately 10 days. The T-tube should remain *in situ* for a further 3 weeks to establish a satisfactory track before removal.

Key point 6

- The differential diagnosis of jaundice in infancy includes inspissated bile syndrome and perforation of the common bile duct.

CHOLELITHIASIS

In the prepubertal child, gallstones are associated with conditions such as chronic haemolysis, cystic fibrosis and ileal resection. The sex incidence is equal and calcium bilirubinate and carbonate are the common constituents of the stones. After puberty, predisposing factors are similar to those found in

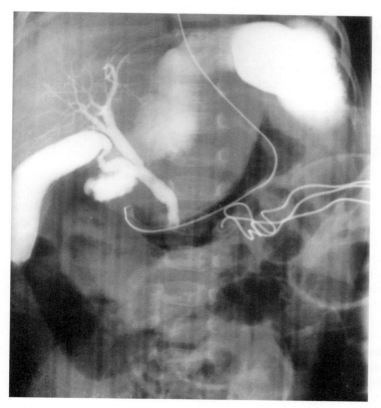

Fig. 4 Operative cholangiogram showing a spontaneous perforation of the common bile duct in a boy 5 weeks of age. Contrast is leaking into the lesser sac.

adults in that there is an increased incidence in girls and cholesterol stones are more common. Stones are frequently asymptomatic in children, and younger children may not localise abdominal pain to the right hypochondrium.

The majority of stones are radiolucent and the diagnosis is usually made with ultrasonography. Antenatal ultrasonography has revealed echogenic foci within the gallbladder during the 3rd trimester, although there are no obvious predisposing factors and they usually disappear spontaneously.[37,38] Stone formation may follow a period of parenteral nutrition but, in the absence of inspissated bile, most remain asymptomatic and few develop complications. Most appear to resolve with the resumption of enteral feeding.[39,40]

The medical treatment of gallstones remains disappointing. The use of ursodeoxycholic acid (UDCA) for 1 year in 15 children with a mean age of 8 years, for example, resulted in the disappearance of the stones in 2 cases but these reappeared later.[41] However, all symptomatic patients did become symptom free.

Laparoscopic cholecystectomy is the definitive treatment of choice for symptomatic gallstones in childhood. A comparison of 29 consecutive open cholecystectomies with 21 laparoscopic operations showed a significantly shorter period of hospitalisation in the laparoscopic group ($P = 0.015$).[42] Interestingly, common bile duct stones were present in 13 (26%) of the 50 children, most of whom had gallstones secondary to sickle cell disease.

Key point 7

- Laparoscopic cholecystectomy is the treatment of choice for gallstones in all age groups.

HEPATIC TUMOURS

Primary liver tumours account for approximately 15% of abdominal tumours in childhood and may be either epithelial or mesenchymal in origin and benign or malignant. Malignancy accounts for nearly two-thirds of these tumours and a logical protocol of investigation is necessary for rapid investigation and treatment. Secondary hepatic tumours, such as neuroblastoma, may also affect this age group.

Most tumours present before 2 years of age and most are treated by resection.

A wide range of liver tumours occurs in paediatric practice, although all of them are very rare. A simple classification of the most frequent types is shown in Table 1.

Paediatric liver tumours have also been associated with a variety of congenital disorders including hemihypertrophy, biliary atresia, polyposis coli, von Gierke's disease, tyrosinaemia, Beckwith's syndrome and congenital malformations of the portal vein.[43]

The commonest presentation is with an asymptomatic abdominal mass. Pain, fever, anorexia and weakness are indicative of advanced disease and metastases are present in approximately 25% at diagnosis.

Table 1 A simple classification of the most frequent types of liver tumours occurring in paediatric practice

Benign	Malignant
Haemangioendothelioma	Hepatoblastoma
Mesenchymal hamartoma	Hepatocellular carcinoma
Adenoma	Mesenchymoma
Focal nodular hyperplasia	Yolk sac tumour
Non-parasitic cysts	Angiosarcoma

Diagnosis is made from clinical examination, biopsy , tumour markers and radiological studies. Hepatoblastoma cells produce proteins which occur normally during embryonic development and the majority of hepatoblastomas (90%) secrete α-fetoprotein. This acts as a sensitive tumour marker reflecting changes in tumour volume and it is, therefore, used for diagnosis and for measuring the response to therapy.

Ultrasonography, computed tomography (CT) and angiography are all useful in staging these tumours. Magnetic resonance imaging (MRI) adds detailed information on vascular and segmental anatomy and is particularly useful in showing the hepatic veins (Fig. 5) and inferior vena cava.[44]

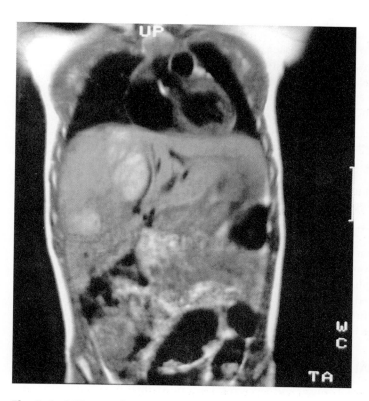

Fig. 5 An MRI scan of a 9-year-old girl. A hepatoblastoma is filling the right half of the liver and displacing the right hepatic vein without invasion.

Tumour resection may include up to 85% of the liver volume without precipitating liver failure, providing the remaining liver is non-cirrhotic. Resection is always performed through a bilateral subcostal incision without entering the chest. Pre-operative chemotherapy is effective in reducing the size of hepatoblastomas by 35–95% and combination chemotherapy and surgery is now mandatory for these malignant tumours.

Transplantation is possible for otherwise irresectable cases; from the limited data available at the moment, the survival rate after transplantation for extensive malignant lesions is greater than 50%.[45]

Key point 8

- Paediatric hepatic tumours commonly present as an asymptomatic mass.

HAEMANGIOENDOTHELIOMA

Hepatic haemangiomata account for approximately 10% of liver masses. Their natural history is similar to that of haemangiomata elsewhere in the body with rapid growth in the first 6 months of life and then gradual resolution. In some cases, however, arterio-venous communications result in severe congestive heart failure which, if untreated, may lead to early death within the first few weeks of life in over 75% of cases.

Hepatic haemangiomata are frequently associated with haemangiomata of the skin and, occasionally, in the gastrointestinal tract or the brain. Over 80% are diagnosed before 6 months of age and the male:female incidence is equal. Investigations include ultrasonography, CT and angiography.

Key point 9

- Hepatic haemangiomata in infancy may cause severe heart failure. Hepatic artery ligation is curative.

Treatment varies according to the severity of symptoms. Steroids may hasten resolution in a minority of cases and segmental resection may be possible for localised lesions. Hepatic artery ligation, first reported in 1967,[46] is now an accepted and effective treatment for diffuse haemangiomata. There were 9 successfully treated cases in a recent series of 11 infants, 3 of whom underwent resection (1 death) and 8 hepatic artery ligation (1 death).[47]

MESENCHYMAL HAMARTOMA

These lesions are benign and account for approximately 6% of primary tumours. Two-thirds present in the first year and almost all before 5 years of age. They are cystic lesions containing either clear fluid or mucoid material and, although they are usually confined to one half of the liver, they may grow to over 2 kg in weight. Histologically there is a mixture of mesodermal and endodermal structure in a connective tissue stroma and bile duct, liver cell, and angiomatous components are typical. These hamartomata are thought to represent a failure of normal development and arise from connective tissue tracts within the fetal liver.

An asymptomatic mass is the commonest presentation, but occasionally patients present with respiratory embarrassment from pressure on the diaphragms. Angiography demonstrates these tumours as relatively avascular structures.

HEPATOBLASTOMA

Hepatoblastoma is the most common malignant hepatic tumour in childhood; but it is rare and occurs with a frequency of approximately 1 case per million children less than 15 years of age per year. This represents 0.8–1.0% of all childhood malignant tumours. Although there is no variation in incidence throughout the world, an increasing incidence has been noted. A relationship with the increased survival of low birth weight infants has been suggested.[48]

A relationship of hepatoblastoma and familial adenomatous polyposis (FAP) is of interest and an investigation of 25 hepatoblastoma children who had a family history of FAP revealed adenomatous lesions in 6 survivors between the ages of 7–25 years. These observations suggest the involvement of a common chromosomal abnormality, perhaps related to chromosome 5.[49,50]

As with other hepatic tumours, an asymptomatic abdominal mass is the commonest presenting feature. Pain may be related to capsular stretching, haemorrhage or tumour infarction and many of the patients are anaemic.

Serum α-fetoprotein is a particularly sensitive tumour marker for hepatoblastoma and the extent of the lesion can be accurately assessed with CT, MRI and angiography. A percutaneous liver biopsy is performed before starting chemotherapy.

Total resection remains the essential treatment for the cure of hepato-blastoma. However, pre-operative chemotherapy is now used routinely except for the occasional small lesion found in a very lateral position in the liver.

Results

The survival results before the refinement of liver resection technique and before the introduction of effective chemotherapy were poor. For example, of 35 hepatoblastomata reported in 1967 only 18 were resectable and the operative mortality was 22%. Only 6 patients (17%) survived for a significant period of time.[51] An operative mortality rate of 22.5% was reported from a collected series of 223 cases in 1975.[52]

Key point 10

- Combination chemotherapy and surgery provides effective treatment for hepatoblastoma.

These figures can be compared with a collected series of cases treated with combined chemotherapy and surgery since 1990, which show resection rates of 72–100% and survival rates of over 66%.[53]

Transplantation is now an alternative treatment for tumours that are too extensive for more conventional surgery. A collected review of transplantation in 18 patients with hepatoblastomata reported tumour recurrence in 6 (33%), and a 2 and 5-year tumour free survival rate of 50%.[45]

Key points for clinical practice

- Early surgery is essential for biliary atresia.

- Portoenterostomy for biliary atresia can result in good bile flow and long-term survival has been proven.

- Jaundice and/or pancreatitis are frequent presentations of choledochal cysts.

- Pancreatitis in childhood may be associated with a common pancreatico-biliary channel.

- Total excision is the treatment of choice for choledochal cysts.

- The differential diagnosis of jaundice in infancy includes inspissated bile syndrome and perforation of the common bile duct.

- Laparoscopic cholecystectomy is the treatment of choice for gallstones in all age groups.

- Paediatric hepatic tumours commonly present as an asymptomatic mass.

- Hepatic haemangiomata may cause severe heart failure. Hepatic artery ligation is curative.

- Combination chemotherapy and surgery provide effective treatment for hepatoblastoma.

References

1. Hays D M, Kimura K. Biliary atresia: the Japanese experience. Cambridge, MA: Harvard University Press, 1980: 20–23.
2. Davenport M, Howard E R. Macroscopic appearance at portoenterostomy – a prognostic variable in biliary atresia. J Pediatr Surg 1996; 31: 1387–1390.
3. Davenport M, Savage M, Mowat A P, Howard E R The biliary atresia-splenic malformation syndrome: an aetiological and prognostic subgroup. Surgery 1993; 113: 662–668.
4. MacGillivray T E, Scott Adzick N. Biliary atresia begins before birth. Pediatr Surg Int 1994; 9: 116-117.
5. Redkar R, Davenport M, Howard E R. Antenatal diagnosis of congenital anomalies of the biliary tract. J Pediatr Surg 1998; 33: 700–704.
6. Parashar K, Taplow M J, McCrae M A. Experimental reovirus type 3-induced murine biliary tract disease. J Pediatr Surg 1992; 27: 843–847.
7. Riepenhoff-Talty M, Schaekel K, Clark H F et al. Group A rotaviruses produce extrahepatic biliary obstruction in orally inoculated newborn mice. Pediatr Res 1993; 33: 394–399.

8. Tan C E L, Moscoso G J, Howard E R, Driver M. Extrahepatic biliary atresia: a first trimester event? Clues from light microscopy and immunohistochemistry. J Pediatr Surg 1994; 29: 808–814.

9. Howard E R. Biliary atresia. In: Blumgart L H. (ed) Surgery of the Liver and Biliary Tract, 2nd edn. Edinburgh: Churchill Livingstone, 1994: 835–852.

10. Mieli-Vergani G, Howard E R, Portmann B, Mowat A P. Late referral for biliary atresia – missed opportunities for effective surgery. Lancet 1989; i: 421–423.

11. Tan C E L, Davenport M, Driver M, Howard E R. Does the morphology of the extrahepatic biliary remnants in biliary atresia influence survival? A review of 205 cases. J Pediatr Surg 1994; 29: 1459–1464.

12. Howard E R, Davenport M. The treatment of biliary atresia in Europe 1969–1995. Tohoku J Exp Med 1997; 181: 75–83.

13. Howard E R. Biliary atresia. In: Stringer M D, Oldham K T, Mouriquand P D E, Howard E R. (eds) Pediatric Surgery and Urology: Long Term Outcomes. London: Saunders, 1998: 402–416.

14. Valayer J. Conventional treatment of biliary atresia: long term results. J Pediatr Surg 1996; 31: 1546–1551.

15. Nio M, Ohi R, Hayashi Y, Endo N, Ibrahim M, Iwami D. Current status of 21 living patients surviving more than 20 years after surgery for biliary atresia. J Pediatr Surg 1996; 31: 381–384.

16. Goss J A, Shackleton C R, Swenson K et al. Orthotopic liver transplantation for congenital biliary atresia: an 11 year single-center experience. Ann Surg 1996; 224: 276–284.

17. Tsardakas E, Robnett A H. Congenital cystic dilatation of the common bile duct: report of 3 cases, analysis of 57 cases and review of the literature. Arch Surg 1956; 72: 311–327.

18. Todani T, Watanabe Y, Narusue M, Tobuchi K, Okajima K. Congenital bile duct cysts: classification, operative procedures and review of 37 cases including cancer arising from choledochal cyst. Am J Surg. 1977; 134: 263–269.

19. Stringer M D, Dhawan A, Davenport M, Mieli-Vergani G, Mowat A P, Howard E R. Choledochal cysts: lessons from a 20 year experience. Arch Dis Child 1995; 73: 528–531.

20. Redkar R, Davenport M, Howard E R. Antenatal diagnosis of congenital anomalies of the biliary tract. J Pediatr Surg 1998; 33: 700–704.

21. Raffensperger J G, Given G Z, Warner R A. Fusiform dilatation of the common bile duct with pancreatitis. J Pediatr Surg 1973; 8: 907–910.

22. Davenport M, Stringer M D, Howard E R. Biliary amylase and congenital choledochal dilatation. J Pediatr Surg 1995; 30: 474–477.

23. Komi N, Takehara H, Kunimoto K, Miyoshi Y, Yagi T. Does the type of anomalous arrangement of pancreaticobiliary ducts influence the surgery and prognosis of choledochal cysts? J Pediatr Surg 1992; 27: 728–731.

24. Misra S P, Dwivedi M. Pancreaticobiliary ductal union. Gut 1990; 31: 1144–1149.

25. Lilly J, Stellin G P, Karrer F M. Forme fruste choledochal cyst. J Pediatr Surg 1985; 20: 449–451.

26. Komi N, Tamura T, Tsuge S, Miyoshi Y, Udaka H, Takehara H. Relation of patient age to premalignant alterations in choledochal cyst epithelium: histochemical and immunohistochemical studies. J Pediatr Surg 1986; 21: 430–433.

27. Shimada K, Yanagisawa J, Nakayama F. Increased lysophosphatidylcholine and pancreatic enzyme content in bile of patients with anomalous pancreaticobiliary junction. Hepatology 1991; 13: 438–444.

28. Sugiyama M, Atomi Y. Anomalous pancreaticobiliary junction without congenital choledochal cyst. Br J Surg 1998; 85: 911–916.

29. Yamashiro Y, Sato M, Hoshino A. Spontaneous perforation of a choledochal cyst. Eur J Pediatr 1982; 138: 193–195.

30. Ando K, Miyano T, Kohno S, Takamizawa S, Lane G. Spontaneous perforation of choledochal cyst: a study of 13 cases. Eur J Pediatr Surg 1998; 8: 23–25.

31. Tan K C, Howard E R. Choledochal cyst: a 14-year surgical experience with 36 patients. Br J Surg 1988; 75: 892–895.

32. Watts D R, Lorenzo G A, Beal J M. Congenital dilatation of the intrahepatic biliary ducts. Arch Surg 1974; 108: 592.

33. Rodgers B M, Hollenbeck J I, Donnelly W H, Talbert J L. Intrahepatic cholestasis with parenteral alimentation. Am J Surg 1976; 131: 149–155.

Recent Advances in Surgery 23

34. Heaton N D, Davenport M, Howard E R. Intraluminal biliary obstruction. Arch Dis Child 1991; 66: 1395–1398.

35. Petterson G. Spontaneous perforation of the common bile duct in infants. Acta Chir Scand 1955; 60: 192–201.

36. Davenport M, Heaton N D, Howard E R. Spontaneous perforation of the bile ducts in infants. Br J Surg 1991; 78: 1068–1070.

37. Brown D L, Teele R L, Doubilet P M et al. Echogenic material in the fetal gallbladder: sonographic and clinical observations. Radiology 1992; 182: 73–76.

38. Stringer M D, Lim P, Cave M, Martinez D, Lilford R J. Fetal gallstones. J Pediatr Surg 1996; 31: 1589–1591.

39. Jacir N N, Anderson K D, Eichelberger M, Guzzetta P C. Cholelithiasis in infancy: resolution of gallstones in three of four infants. J Pediatr Surg 1986; 21: 567–569.

40. St-Vil D, Yazbeck S, Luks F I, Hancock B J, Filiatrault D, Youssef S. Cholelithiasis in newborns and infants. J Pediatr Surg 1992; 27: 1305–1307.

41. Gamba P G, Zancan L, Midrio P et al. Is there a place for medical treatment in children with gallstones? J Pediatr Surg 1997; 32: 476–478.

42. Al Salem A H, Qaisaruddin S, Al-Abkari H, Nourallah H, Yassin Y M, Varma K K. Laparoscopic versus open cholecystectomy in children. Pediatr Surg Int 1997; 12: 587–590.

43. Howard E R, Heaton N D. Benign and malignant hepatic tumours. In: Howard E R. (ed) Surgery of Liver Disease in Children. Oxford: Butterworth-Heinemann, 1991: 126–142.

44. Finn J P, Hall-Craggs M A, Dicks-Mireaux C et al. Primary malignant liver tumours in childhood: assessment and resectability with high-field MR and comparison with CT. Pediatr Radiol 1990; 21: 34–38.

45. Penn I. Hepatic transplantation for primary and metastatic cancers of the liver. Surgery 1991; 110: 726–735.

46. DeLorimer A A, Simpson E B, Baum R S, Carlsson E. Hepatic artery ligation for hepatic hemangiomatosis. N Engl J Med 1967; 277: 333–337.

47. Davenport M, Hansen L, Heaton N D, Howard E R. Haemangioendothelioma of the liver in infants. J Pediatr Surg 1995; 30: 44–48.

48. Ross J A, Gurney J G. Hepatoblastoma incidence in the United States from 1973 to 1992. Med Pediatr Oncol 1998; 30: 141–142.

49. Garber J E, Li F P, Kingston J E et al. Hepatoblastoma and familial adenomatous polyposis. Report of two cases. Dis Colon Rectum. 1992; 35: 373–374.

50. Phillips M, Dicks-Mireaux, Kingston M et al. Hepatoblastoma and polyposis coli (familial adenomatous polyposis). Med Pediatr Oncol 1989; 17: 441–447.

51. Ishak K G, Glunz P R. Hepatoblastoma and hepatocarcinoma in infancy and childhood. Cancer 1967; 20: 396–422.

52. Exelby P R, Filler R M, Grosfield J L. Liver tumours in children in particular reference to hepatoblastoma and hepatocellular carcinoma: American Academy of Pediatrics Surgical Section Survey – 1974. J Pediatr Surg 1975; 10: 329–337.

53. Howard E R, Ruers T J. Hepatobiliary malignancy in childhood. In: Terblanche J. (ed) Hepatobiliary Malignancy. London: Edward Arnold, 1994: 251–170.

Mohammad Bashar Izzat Loay S. Kabbani
Gianni D. Angelini

CHAPTER

8

Minimal-access and minimally invasive cardiac surgery

The significance of trauma of the surgical incision and its associated morbidity has become widely appreciated in the various surgical specialties. Cardiac surgery, however, is the last of these to attempt to minimize the trauma of access, and this is largely due to the inherent complexities of cardiac operations.[1] Until recently, therefore, median sternotomy has remained the standard approach for most open-heart procedures because it provides easy exposure of the entire heart and allows for the various cardiopulmonary bypass and myocardial protection techniques. The past 3 years, however, have witnessed the introduction of alternative incisions to median sternotomy, and a variety of heart operations have been performed successfully using these new approaches.[2] Simultaneously, advances were being achieved in avoiding the use of cardiopulmonary bypass and its associated morbidity during coronary revascularization procedures (the so-called 'off-pump' technique). In due course, the combination of both 'minimal-access' and 'off-pump' concepts has formed the basis for attempting off-pump coronary revascularization through small incisions.[1]

It is fitting at the beginning to define 'minimally-invasive' and 'minimal access' surgical techniques. Minimizing the 'invasiveness' of surgery implies reducing the peri-operative morbidity defined by measures of clinical outcome in comparison to conventional techniques. In general surgery, the trauma of the surgical incision is thought to be a principal cause of postoperative pain

Mr Mohammad Bashar Izzat MD MS FRCS(CTh), Consultant Cardiothoracic Surgeon, Damascus University Cardiovascular Surgical Center, Damascus, Syria (correspondence to Dr M.B. Izzat, PO Box 33831, Damascus, Syria)

Dr Loay S. Kabbani MD, Clinical Fellow in Cardiac Surgery, Damascus University Cardiovascular Surgical Center, Damascus, Syria

Prof. Gianni D. Angelini MD MCh FRCS, British Heart Foundation Professor of Cardiac Surgery, Bristol Heart Institute, University of Bristol, Bristol BS2 8HW, UK

and morbidity; so much so that minimizing invasiveness has become synonymous with using small incisions (i.e. minimizing access). In the specific context of heart operations, however, extracorporeal circulation is another significant cause of patient morbidity. Hence, avoiding the use of cardiopulmonary bypass, regardless of the type of surgical incision, is another minimally invasive approach in cardiac surgery.[3,4]

This article summarizes the recent advances in minimal-access and minimally invasive cardiac surgery.

MINIMAL-ACCESS CARDIAC SURGERY

A variety of alternative incisions to median sternotomy have been introduced over the past 3 years, many of which remain investigational, and a few have already been abandoned.[2] Nevertheless, experience to-date has already shown that postoperative pain may be reduced and patient recovery enhanced by avoiding the trauma of median sternotomy in some cardiac operations.[5]

Currently employed minimal-access approaches to heart operations can be broadly classified into: (i) direct-vision techniques through limited incisions; and (ii) video-assisted approaches using endoscopic methods.

DIRECT-VISION SURGERY THROUGH LIMITED INCISIONS

Early in the development of minimal-access cardiac surgery, a right parasternal incision was employed to attain surgical access to heart chambers which compares to that achieved by median sternotomy.[6–8] This incision extends from the lower edge of the second costal cartilage to the superior edge of the fifth costal cartilage (Fig. 1). By excising the third and fourth right costal cartilages and incising the pericardium longitudinally, the ascending aorta and right atrium are exposed. Direct cannulation of the aorta and the superior and

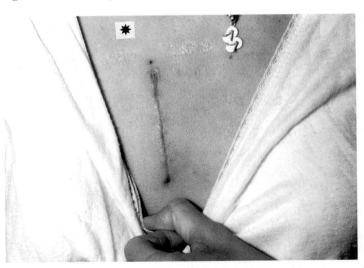

Fig. 1 Skin incision for a right parasternal approach used for closure of atrial septal defect. *Second intercostal space.

inferior vena cava is feasible, and aortic and/or mitral valve procedures as well as repair of atrial septal defects can be performed in the standard fashion. Use of this incision has been shown to be associated with reduced postoperative pain and morbidity.[6–8] However, late chest wall deformity, the possibility of lung herniation through the defect in the chest wall, as well as the introduction of better alternative incisions led to the abandoning of this approach.[2]

At present, the partial sternotomy incision is the most commonly used minimal-access approach for intra-cardiac operations. It has many of the advantages of median sternotomy; the incision is easily opened and closed, provides excellent access, allows for standard cardiopulmonary bypass techniques, and can be easily converted to full sternotomy in troublesome cases.[5,9,10] With an **upper** partial sternotomy, the sternum is split from the sternal notch to the level of the third intercostal space. The split is then either extended as a 'T' into the third intercostal space on either side or carried into the fourth right intercostal space in a 'hockey-stick' fashion. The ascending aorta and most of the right atrium are well exposed (Fig. 2), and cannulation for cardiopulmonary bypass is performed directly through the incision. Aortic

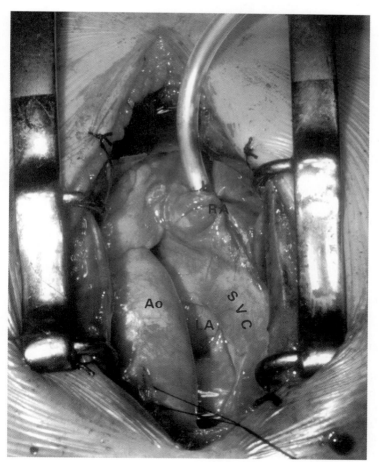

Fig. 2 Operative view of an upper mini-sternotomy incision. The aorta (Ao), superior vena cava (SVC), right atrium (RA) and roof of left atrium (LA) are well exposed.

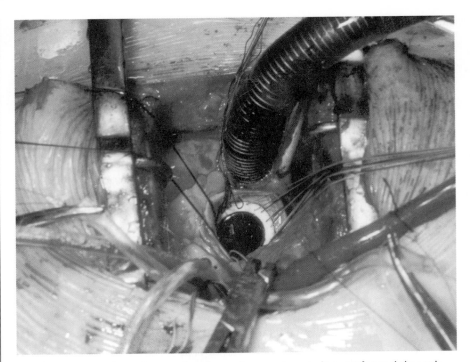

Fig. 3 Operative view of an aortic valve replacement procedure performed through an upper mini-sternotomy. The aorta and right atrial appendage were cannulated directly through the incision, and a mechanical bileaflet valve prosthesis is being implanted.

and mitral valve procedures are performed in the standard fashion (Fig. 3).[5,9,10] Alternatively, a **lower** partial sternotomy incision can be used, dividing the sternum from the xiphoid process up to the level of the second rib, and terminating the sternal split into the left 2nd intercostal space. Cannulation for cardiopulmonary bypass can also be performed directly through the incision. Coronary artery bypass grafting to the left anterior descending and right coronary arteries can be performed through this incision, with or without cardiopulmonary bypass support.[11] We have also used this incision for atrial septal defect closure[7] and to perform valve replacements in patients with permanent tracheostomies to avoid the risk of life-threatening sternal wound infection.

Clinical experience with minimal access direct-vision surgery

The value of minimal access cardiac surgery as described above is measured by the overall results it achieves for both surgeons and patients.[2] On both counts, minimizing access has been advantageous in clinical experience. For the surgeon, opening and closing the chest is easier and faster,[8] and mediastinal blood loss is significantly reduced, probably because mediastinal dissection is minimized.[5] These patients are extubated, discharged from hospital, and resume normal activities earlier than those who undergo the conventional operation. Postoperative pain is also reported to be reduced, both in hospital and after discharge.[5,8–10] Needless to say, the smaller incision is cosmetically more acceptable.[12] Another potential advantage of the minimal access approach is that the pericardium is not fully opened; hence re-operations should be easier and safer.

The potential disadvantages of these procedures should be considered as well. One concern relates to the stability of the chest wall after the excision of multiple costal cartilages in the right para-sternal approach. Paradoxical motion of the chest wall, particularly during coughing, has been observed in most patients, and this is the principal reason for the reduced popularity of this approach. Overall, however, it is clear from the clinical experience at hand that the same quality of operations can be performed through less traumatic and better cosmetic incisions at a lower overall cost, achieving many of the good goals of managed care.[12]

VIDEO-ASSISTED THORACOSCOPIC CARDIAC SURGERY

Video-assistance is well recognized as the backbone of minimal-access and endoscopic procedures. At present, however, video-assistance remains limited to a few applications in cardiac surgery due to the complexities of cardiac procedures. For example, performing coronary anastomoses endoscopically, albeit already done in animal laboratories, has not yet been possible in the clinical setting. The only established role for the video-assisted technique at present is in thoracoscopic mitral valve surgery, but it can also be used for harvesting the internal mammary artery in preparation for the minimally invasive direct coronary artery bypass (MIDCAB) procedure (see below).

Video-assisted mitral valve surgery can be performed through the so-called 'micro-mitral' technique.[13] With this method, cardiopulmonary bypass perfusion is achieved through femoral vessel cannulation, and aortic occlusion by means of a special trans-thoracic aortic cross-clamp. A 6 cm right infra-mammary incision is made, and a short segment of the 4th rib is resected. Conventional surgical instruments are introduced through this manipulation incision, and the mitral valve procedure is performed using thoracoscopic display, which projects a magnified view of high resolution on the monitor screen. We have performed both mitral valve repair and replacement procedures successfully with this technique.

An alternative technique is the Port-Access method (Heartport, Inc., Redwood City, CA, USA).[14] This cardiopulmonary bypass cannulation system uses a specially designed femoral arterial cannula with a side arm for placement of an endo-aortic balloon, which is positioned in the ascending aorta. Inflating the balloon will occlude the ascending aorta, and cardioplegic solution is then delivered antegradely through its lumen for myocardial protection. The mitral valve procedure (repair or replacement) is performed through a small manipulation incision under video-guidance with the use of special endoscopic instruments.[14]

Clinical experience with video-assisted thoracoscopic mitral valve surgery

Reports on the early clinical experience with thoracoscopic mitral valve surgery are already available, and indicate that these techniques may benefit patients through reduced intensive care unit stay, lower blood transfusion requirement, less postoperative discomfort and earlier hospital discharge.[13,14] These positive features, however, have been challenged and the safety of these techniques has been called into question. Both operative and extracorporeal perfusion times tend to be prolonged, and the new technical challenges presented by endoscopic surgery have been an added burden. Nevertheless, it is likely that broader experience with video assistance should diminish these concerns and, indeed, recent reports have presented extracorporeal perfusion times approximating those associated with conventional surgery.

Of particular concern is the number of serious complications that occurred using the Port-Access techniques. There were cases of acute aortic dissection, likely to have been caused by intimal dissection induced by the guide wire and retrograde aortic perfusion, as well as local complications at the groin and ischaemic complications of the leg. A range of other potential complications deserve consideration as well, such as flushing atheromatous debris from the descending aorta into the cerebral circulation, proximal balloon displacement with damage to the aortic valve, or distal balloon displacement obstructing the brachiocephalic trunk.[2,14]

Clearly, the design and instrumentation of current systems needs further improvement to enhance their safety and efficacy. Present systems and techniques, however, are a transitory step in the evolution of minimal access cardiac surgery. What is certain at present is that this development is dependent on the broader use of video-assisted techniques, the benefits of which are being recognized rapidly by cardiac surgeons world-wide.

CORONARY REVASCULARIZATION WITHOUT CARDIOPULMONARY BYPASS

Coronary artery bypass grafting without cardiopulmonary bypass is a surgical strategy that has gained increasing popularity for a variety of reasons, foremost among which is the increasing operative risk of patients referred for operation.[15,16] These patients are not only older but are also affected by several co-morbid states more often than candidates seen a decade ago. Such patients will poorly tolerate the side effects of hypotensive non-pulsatile extracorporeal perfusion and systemic cooling. It has been recognized that no notable decrease in the morbidity of coronary artery surgery is likely, particularly in this high risk group of patients, unless use of cardiopulmonary bypass can be avoided.[1,15,16]

CORONARY REVASCULARIZATION THROUGH MEDIAN STERNOTOMY

The principal challenge during off-pump coronary artery grafting is to perform accurate micro-vascular anastomoses to the constantly moving targeted coronary arteries. Early attempts for off-pump grafting were largely limited to grafting the left anterior descending coronary artery due to its technical easiness; however, with the development of techniques and devices that can effectively stabilize the various coronary arteries, this was rapidly extended to multivessel revascularization.[17–19] At present, over 60% of all patients with multi-vessel coronary artery disease can be completely revascularized without the use of cardiopulmonary bypass.

Clinical experience with off-pump grafting in patients with indicators of high peri-operative risk has demonstrated significant improvements in early awakening, duration of mechanical ventilation, amount of postoperative bleeding and need for blood transfusion, length of intensive care unit stay and total hospital stay.[16,19] Early concerns about the accuracy of coronary grafting without cardiopulmonary bypass were alleviated by several studies using postoperative angiography which have demonstrated that technically correct anastomoses can be repeatedly and reliably performed on the beating heart.[20–22]

Early experience with coronary revascularization without cardiopulmonary bypass has been very encouraging, and is now the technique of choice for routine coronary grafting in many centres. Moreover, the advent of this technique has opened the door to accepting patients from several risk categories for coronary revascularization.

SINGLE VESSEL GRAFTING THROUGH A MINI-THORACOTOMY

Grafting the left anterior descending coronary artery (LAD) with the left internal mammary artery (LIMA) can be performed successfully via a left anterior mini-thoracotomy, a technique now known as minimally invasive direct coronary artery bypass (MIDCAB).[23] With this technique, a 6 cm mini-thoracotomy incision is made in the 4th left intercostal space, the LIMA is mobilized from its bed, either under direct vision or with thoracoscopic assistance,[24] and is then grafted to the LAD without the use of cardiopulmonary bypass (Fig. 4). This technique can also be applied to grafting the right coronary artery with the right internal mammary artery.

Significant experience already exists with MIDCAB, with an impressive 95% early patency rate presented in the largest published series.[25] With MIDCAB, the trauma of access is minimal, patient comfort is high and hospital stay is limited to 2–3 days.

Although MIDCAB has been used predominantly in patients with single vessel disease, its use was also extended to patients with multiple vessel disease in whom conventional coronary bypass surgery is associated with increased risk because of various associated medical conditions.[26] This application is based on the favourable natural history of patients with multivessel coronary artery disease but with patent LIMA to LAD grafts. In this way, MIDCAB offers a low risk palliative operation. Moreover, in selected cases, the protection conferred by a patent LIMA to LAD graft can allow revascularization to be extended further at a second stage with percutaneous balloon angioplasty of other coronary arteries.[27–28]

THE FUTURE

It is not possible to tell what form cardiac surgery practice will take in 5 years' time. It is likely that coronary artery grafting without cardiopulmonary bypass will become the procedure of choice for coronary revascularization. Gradually,

Minimal-access and minimally invasive cardiac surgery

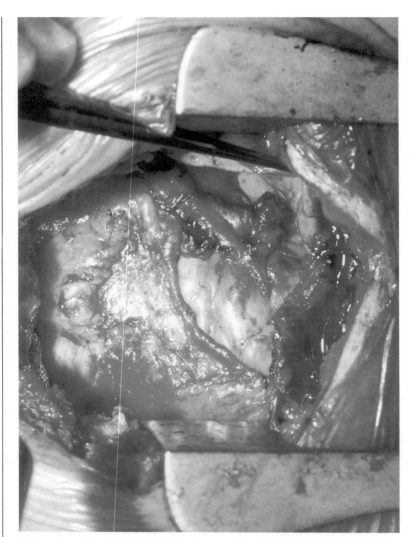

Fig. 4 Operative view upon completion of a MIDCAB procedure. The left internal mammary artery was anastomosed to the left anterior descending coronary artery. The star marks the anastomosis. The dotted line marks the internal mammary artery. The left ventricle is visible through a small window in the pericardium.

more intra-cardiac operative procedures will be performed using video-assisted techniques; however it is likely that most cardiac procedures will continue to be performed through median sternotomy until advanced (and possibly computer-assisted) endoscopic techniques are developed and refined.

There is little doubt already that the face of cardiac surgery has been changed forever by the advent of the new minimal-access and minimally invasive techniques. The potential for decreased complication rates, shorter hospital stay and lower cost of care has created broad interest.[29,30] Moreover, the massive publicity which has accompanied the realization that the 'mutilation' of sternotomy is no longer an essential part of heart operations is an important factor which is likely to drive the development of minimal access approaches. The 'public demand' scenario that has led laparoscopic cholecystectomy to become the standard surgical approach appears to be repeating itself in cardiac surgery.

In our opinion, the concepts of minimal-access and minimally invasive heart surgery are advantageous and deserve further investigation and development. The safety of these innovative approaches, however, is a pressing issue which must be addressed continuously in as much as surgical precision and clinical outcome should not be sacrificed for the pledge of benefits ascribed to reduced short-term morbidity. Certainly, newly developed therapeutic modalities must at least duplicate the efficacy and safety of conventional surgical techniques.

Key points for clinical practice

- Avoiding the use of the extracorporeal circulation (minimal invasion) rather than small incision (minimal access) is the main goal of the cardiac surgeon.

- Coronary artery bypass grafting without cardiopulmonary bypass is likely to become routine in the next few years.

References

1. Izzat M B, Yim A P C. Minimally invasive cardiac surgery, a fleeting fancy or a lasting prospect? [Editorial] Int J Cardiol 1997; 59: 223–225.
2. Izzat M B, Yim A P C. Intracardiac surgery. In: Cohn RG, Mack MJ, Fonger JD, Landerneau RJ (eds) Minimally Invasive Cardiac Surgery. St Louis, MO: QMP Publishers, 1999; 257–264.
3. Izzat M B, Yim A P C. To know chalk from cheese [Editorial]. J Card Surg 1997; 12: 360–361.
4. Izzat M B, Calafiore A M, Yim A P C. What's in a name? [Editorial] Heart Surg Forum 1998; 1: 99–100.
5. Izzat M B, Yim A P C, El-Zufari M H, Khow K S. Upper 'T' mini-sternotomy for aortic valve operations. Chest 1998; 114: 291–294.
6. Cosgrove D M, Sabik J F. Minimally invasive approach for aortic valve operations. Ann Thorac Surg 1996; 62: 596–597.
7. Izzat M B, Yim A P C, El-Zufari M H. Limited access atrial septal defect closure and the evolution of minimally invasive surgery. Ann Thorac Cardiovasc Surg 1998; 4: 56–58.
8. Cosgrove D M, Sabik J F, Navia J L. Minimally invasive valve operations. Ann Thorac Surg 1998; 65: 1535–1539.
9. Gundry S R, Shattuck O H, Razzouk A J, del Rio M J, Sardari F F, Bailey L L. Facile minimally invasive cardiac surgery via ministernotomy. Ann Thorac Surg 1998; 65: 1100–1104.
10. Izzat M B, Wan S, Wan I Y P, Khaw K, Yim A P C. Aortic valve replacement through mini-sternotomy in a patient with osteogenesis imperfecta. Ann Thorac Surg 1999; 67: 1171–1173.
11. Arom K V, Emery R W, Nicoloff D M. Mini-sternotomy for coronary artery bypass grafting. Ann Thorac Surg 1996; 61: 1271–1272.
12. Cohn L H, Adams D H, Couper G S et al. Minimally invasive cardiac valve surgery improves patient satisfaction while reducing costs of cardiac valve replacement and repair. Ann Surg 1997; 226: 421–428.

13. Chitwood W R, Wixon C L, Elbeery J R, Moran J F, Chapman W H H, Lust R M. Video-assisted minimally invasive mitral valve surgery. J Thorac Cardiovasc Surg 1997; 114: 773–782.

14. Mohr F W, Falk V, Diegeler A, Walther , van Son J A M, Autschbach R. Minimally invasive port-access mitral valve surgery. J Thorac Cardiovasc Surg 1998; 115: 567–576.

15. Bryan A J, Angelini G D. Minimal access coronary artery surgery [Editorial]. Heart 1997; 77: 307–308.

16. Buffolo E, de Andrade J C S, Branco J N R, Teles C A, Aguiar L F, Gomes W J. Coronary artery bypass grafting without cardiopulmonary bypass. Ann Thorac Surg 1996; 61: 63–66.

17. Izzat M B, Yim A P C. Cardiac stabilizer for minimally invasive direct coronary artery bypass. Ann Thorac Surg 1997; 64: 570–571.

18. Lucchetti V, Angelini G D. An inexpensive method of heart stabilization during coronary artery operations without cardiopulmonary bypass. Ann Thorac Surg 1998; 65: 1477–1478.

19. Jansen E W L, Borst C, Lahpor J R et al. Coronary artery bypass grafting without cardiopulmonary bypass using the Octopus method: results in the first one hundred patients. J Thorac Cardiovasc Surg 1998; 116: 60–67.

20. Izzat M B, Yim A P C. Didn't they do well? [Editorial] Ann Thorac Surg 1997; 64: 1–2.

21. Izzat M B, Yim A P C. MIDCAB: lessons learned from routine 'on-table' angiography. Ann Thorac Surg 1997; 64: 1872–1874.

22. Izzat M B, Yim A P C. Trouble shooting in minimally invasive direct coronary artery bypass. Lancet 1997; 350: 665–666.

23. Calafiore A M, Di Giammarco G, Teodori G et al. Left anterior descending coronary artery grafting via left anterior small thoracotomy without cardiopulmonary bypass. Ann Thorac Surg 1996; 61: 1658–1665.

24. Izzat M B, Yim A P C. Video-assisted internal mammary artery mobilisation for minimally invasive coronary artery bypass. Eur J Cardiothorac Surg 1997; 12: 811–812.

25. Calafiore A M, Di Giammarco G, Teodori G et al. Midterm results after minimally invasive coronary surgery (LAST operation). J Thorac Cardiovasc Surg 1998; 115: 763–771.

26. Izzat M B, Yim A P C. Minimally invasive LAD revascularization in high-risk patients with three-vessel coronary artery disease. Int J Cardiol 1997; 62 (Suppl. 1): S101–S104.

27. Angelini G D, Wilde P, Salerno T A, Bosco G, Calafiore A M. Integrated left small thoracotomy and angioplasty for multivessel coronary artery revascularisation. Lancet 1996; 347: 757–758.

28. Izzat M B, Yim A P C, Mehta D et al. Staged minimally invasive direct coronary artery bypass and percutaneous angioplasty for multivessel coronary artery disease. Int J Cardiol 1997; 62 (Suppl. 1): S105–S109.

29. Calafiore A M, Angelini G D, Bergsland J, Salerno T A. Minimally invasive coronary artery bypass grafting. Ann Thorac Surg 1996; 62: 1545–1548.

30. Treasure T. Minimal access surgery. Heart 1997; 77: 304–306.

John N. Baxter

Recent advances in bariatric surgery

In this non-systematic review of recent advances in bariatric surgery, I shall arbitrarily define 'recent' as within the last 5 years, but what represents an advance is much more difficult to define. Much of the published literature in the last 5 years needs validation before its value as new knowledge can be assessed. What really is an advance takes time and experience to recognise.

For the purposes of this review, morbid obesity is defined as a body mass index (BMI) of equal to, or greater than, 40 kg/m^2. The exact prevalence of morbid obesity in the UK is not known, but probably equates to that of the US where it has been estimated to be around 1% of the population.

The need for obesity surgery may be expected to eventually disappear when all the pathophysiological events causing morbid obesity have been identified and non-surgical treatments have been found for them. Although there is increasing research in obesity, there is still a paucity when compared to research in other common diseases. Despite this, there have been 20 chromosomes identified containing genes (10 autosomal dominant) which are thought to be responsible for obesity. Unravelling how all these genes interact is only in its infancy but will, in the fullness of time, provide insights into the molecular management of this condition. The disease of morbid obesity has a genetic landscape which is acted on by medical, lifestyle and psychological factors which interact to decide the final obesity phenotype.

There is a dearth of good studies of the psychopathology of morbid obesity, much of that which is published being contradictory. A study from California of over 1000 morbidly obese patients has suggested that these patients have excessive somatization, anxiety and depression but not psychoses.[1] The authors argue cogently for adequate counselling for these patients as part of their surgical management programme. Counselling and use of self-help groups are thought to be helpful in the long-term management of morbid obesity after operation but there is a lack of data confirming this. Clearly,

Prof. J.N. Baxter MD FRACS FRCSE FRCSG, Professor of Surgery, University of Wales, Swansea and Honorary Consultant Surgeon, Department of Surgery, Morriston Hospital, Swansea SA6 6NL, UK

surgery for the morbidly obese can never be curative but it ameliorates lifestyle and psychological variables which allows the condition to improve.

THE CASE FOR OBESITY SURGERY

One of the biggest disappointments on reviewing the literature is the lack of research on providing a sound and robust case for the value of obesity surgery. It is generally recognised that obesity surgery is not a cosmetic procedure but is carried out to ameliorate the co-morbid factors described in Table 1. Obesity surgery is the only treatment that provides effective weight loss and long-term weight management in morbidly obese patients. However, continuing need for proof of efficacy is always needed. Despite two US National Institutes of

Table 1 Co-morbidity from morbid obesity

Diabetes mellitus (Type II)
High blood pressure
Dyslipidaemia
Obstructive sleep apnoea
Venous and lymphatic stasis
Osteoarthritis
Decreased mobility
Increased cancer risk (endometrium, prostate, breast, colorectal, cervix, ovary)
Increased risk of cardiac and cerebral vascular events
Chronic respiratory hypoventilation (Pickwickian syndrome)
Hypertrophic cardiomyopathy
Pseudotumour cerebri (idiopathic intracranial hypertension)
Poor quality of life
Increased neuroses
Chronic cholecystitis
Thromboembolic disease
Urinary stress incontinence
Gastro-oesophageal reflux disease
Obesity related pulmonary hypertension
Hernia

Health consensus statements[2] and one recent expert report in the UK[3] suggesting that obesity surgery should be performed more often, there is still a prevalent view that obesity surgery is of low priority and of doubtful value. Moreover, many surgeons feel that obesity is the fault of the patient. The ignorance surrounding this prejudice is astounding. Whilst many surgeons in the UK might potentially be interested in performing obesity surgery, the pressures on the health service result in relegation of obesity surgery to a low priority. A recent survey of obesity surgeons in the UK revealed a very low incidence of obesity procedures in the UK with only 23 surgeons performing any obesity surgery.[4] Many of these surgeons only performed occasional operations.

It is generally agreed by bariatric surgeons that society has to recognise that morbidly obese patients should be seen as victims, not perpetrators, of their incurable disease. Until then, morbidly obesity is the last true bastion of prejudice.[5] Given the cost to society for the morbidity of these patients, it needs to be recognised that morbid obesity is a national health crisis about which little is being done. It has been conservatively estimated that the health-care costs arising from treating all grades of obesity related disorders costs the National Health Service £2 billion annually.

Key point 1

- Prejudice against bariatric surgery is still rife.

Surveys of the efficacy of obesity surgery usually involve descriptions of weight loss following the procedure. Usually this is represented as reduction of BMI from baseline values. An alternative approach is to decide what is the target weight loss to be gained from surgery (usually loss of 50% of excess weight) and see if this is achieved. There is general consensus that obesity surgery is highly effective in reducing BMI or taking greater than 50% of excess body weight off. What is not readily appreciated is that the aim of obesity surgery is not necessarily to approach the ideal body weight for a given individual but to alleviate or 'cure' the co-morbidity which these patients suffer. The weight loss required to improve co-morbidity is much less than usually appreciated and almost certainly is well above ideal body weight. There is some evidence that as little as 10–20% of excess weight reduction may reduce risk factors for co-morbidity to reasonable levels. More studies are needed to examine the definition of success from surgery not only on the basis of actual weight loss but in the prevention, reduction or improvement in co-morbidity.

Key point 2

- Public and health care provider awareness of the cost-effectiveness of bariatric surgery needs to be emphasised.

In one study, it was found that much of the perceived improvement after bariatric surgery was related to the improved mental and physical health rather than actual weight lost.[6] Furthermore, these authors reported that, in these patients, an average of 5.7 years after surgery there was no relationship between presence or absence of presurgical psychiatric diagnosis and weight loss. In another study, patient satisfaction was high after surgery irrespective of which surgical procedure was performed.[7] Perhaps the best quality of life study so far is that from Sweden, where 102 operated patients were followed up for 1.5–5.5 years after vertical banded gastroplasty (VBG) and matched with a cohort of similar operated patients for cholecystectomy. There was a clear improvement in quality of life with gastroplasty having caused a profound change in the patients' lives compared with cholecystectomy patients.[8]

A further study from Germany has also demonstrated an amelioration in metabolic parameters (trigylcerides, insulin, HDL, cholesterol) in 75% of patients after silastic ring vertical gastroplasty.[9] In a similar study from Leeds, patients after a non-banded gastroplasty were apparently cured of type 2 diabetes, and had amelioration of their dyslipidaemia.[10] Furthermore, the same group also reported that, after a partial ileal resection along with a gastroplasty, there is improved control of hypercholesterolaemia.[11] Pories has reported that gastric bypass provides long-term control of non-insulin-dependent diabetes mellitus (NIDDM) with 83% of patients with NIDDM and 99% of patients with glucose impairment maintaining normal levels of glucose, glycosylated haemoglobin and insulin following surgery.[12] He suggested that the antidiabetic effect of surgery appeared to be due primarily to a reduction in caloric intake, suggesting that insulin resistance is a secondary protective effect rather than the initial lesion. A small study of patients after VBG reported loss of left ventricular mass which would hopefully translate to a decrease in overall cardiac risk.[13] Another study from Sweden concluded that after gastroplasty there is improvement in left ventricular filling with improved effects on left ventricular ejection fraction.[14] The Swedish Obesity Subjects (SOS) study, when it finally reports, is going to have the biggest impact on obesity surgery in the next decade. In this study, 2000 patients, after receiving some form of bariatric surgery, are being followed alongside a matched control cohort of conservatively treated patients. Although the study is still accruing patients, it is not far from completion and there is currently a 95% 2-year follow-up. Some of the preliminary data so far published from this study have revealed dramatic improvements in health related quality of life,[15] left ventricular mass, blood pressure, glucose and lipid profiles after surgery compared with controls.

Key point 3

- The Swedish Obesity Subjects study will have an enormous impact on the role of bariatric surgery when the study is fully reported.

SELECTION FOR SURGERY

The International Federation for Surgery of Obesity has recently confirmed the criteria for selection for surgery (Table 2). Most obesity surgeons find that a multidisciplinary team provides better assessment and support for the patient. Booklets should be available giving detailed advice about the type of surgery and its effects, complications and success rate. A dietician, with a special interest in obesity surgery, has a particularly vital role in diet counselling. The surgeon needs to have a physician examine the patient for general fitness and to exclude any endocrine abnormalities. Some multidisciplinary teams include a psychiatrist or psychologist to help in excluding unsuitable patients and also for a counselling role. Despite a feeling that multidisciplinary teams are

Table 2 Criteria for surgery

BMI > 40 kg/m^2
BMI 35–40 kg/m^2 with co-morbid condition improved by weight loss
Age 18–55 years
Fit for surgery
Minimum 5 years' morbid obesity
Failed conservative treatment
No alcoholism or psychosis
Agrees to life-long follow-up

necessary for proper assessment and management of these patients, there are no publications validating this approach.

According to one group of clinicians, if the patient is destined for a gastric bypass there is no need to do any barium studies to exclude concurrent upper gastrointestinal disease.[16] In contrast, another group has reported that, prior to their patients receiving a VBG, a pre-operative gastroscopy has revealed peptic lesions in 37% of patients – a very high incidence.[17] Although difficult to reconcile these two opposing views, it is probable that barium studies are of lower sensitivity and thus endoscopy should probably be performed pre-operatively, although this is by no means a widespread practice. Further studies addressing this question need to be carried out.

The anaesthetist must also assess the patient's fitness for surgery. There is a dearth of good publications on the anaesthetic implications of surgery for morbid obesity. A recent report has demonstrated that, in morbidly obese patients' functional residual capacity, total respiratory compliance is decreased whilst total respiratory system resistance is increased.[18] Furthermore, they also demonstrated that oxygenation index is decreased and the total work of breathing is increased. A Belgian group has shown that a pneumoperitoneum causes significant changes in pulmonary mechanics with a decrease in respiratory compliance and an increase in peak and plateau airway pressures but no change in arterial oxygen saturation.[19] Unfortunately, they did not prospectively compare them to a control population of non-obese or open operation patients. They did suggest, however, that, compared with historical data, morbidly obese patients appear to paradoxically tolerate the pneumoperitoneum better than non-obese patients. The same group of workers in another report suggest that morbidly obese patients experience less haemodynamic changes than non-obese patients with no fall in cardiac output.[20]

It is often questioned whether super-obese patients (BMI > 50 kg/m^2) have a better or worse outcome following obesity surgery. A group from Florida has reported that, after a variety of surgical procedures, 53% of superobese patients lose in excess of 50% of excess weight compared with 71% in the morbidly obese group.[21] Although superobese patients have greater absolute weight loss, they found that morbidly obese patients do better in the long-term.

It is important to remember that, after malabsorption procedures, oral contraceptive medication may not be absorbed so other means of contraception may be advisable. It is generally agreed that pregnancy should be delayed until weight has stabilised after obesity surgery. Vitamin and mineral supplementation is important, viz. iron, calcium, folate, vitamin B$_{12}$ and vitamin A.[22]

The bariatric surgeon should be in close liaison with the obstetrician during a planned pregnancy, since obstetricians are often unaware of the physiological derangements that might ensue in these patients.[22] Another report has highlighted that morbidly obese patients were more likely to experience pregnancy related complications, such as diabetes, hypertension, pre-eclampsia, fetal distress and caesarean section.[23] What has not been reported is the outcome of planned pregnancy in morbidly obese patients after surgically induced weight loss.

All bariatric surgeons would like to know what predictors there are for a poor outcome following surgery, since a variable weight gain nearly always occurs at some time following the nadir of weight loss. A literature review from one group has suggested that binge eating behaviour before surgery may result in an adverse outcome.[24]

Key point 4

- Bariatric surgery should only be carried out within the context of an obesity team.

Key point 5

- Good long-term audit of surgical results needs to be carried out.

OPERATIONS FOR OBESITY

OVERVIEW

This subject has been widely reviewed elsewhere,[25] and was described in *Recent Advances in Surgery*. However, the last 5 years have seen an explosion in laparoscopic procedures such that many procedures may now be performed either as open surgery or laparoscopically. Greater than average laparoscopic skills are required for the more complex procedures, such as VBG or gastric bypass (GBP), which renders them unsuitable for many bariatric surgeons. There is a confusing array of procedures currently available which generally represents the lack of consensus and bias of individual surgeons. Unfortunately, no randomised studies have been performed in the last 5 years to compare procedures. The International Bariatric Surgery Register which has been set up to encourage bariatric surgeons to enter their data and thus allow them to compare their performance with other surgeons last reported in 1997. They have reported on 14,641 patients from over 50 surgeons which has provided little useful data because of the self-selecting nature of the reporting system (see web site).[26] The cost for joining the register is also prohibitively high for many surgeons.

Figure 1 gives an outline of the current surgical procedures that are available. The time honoured argument of what is better – a gastric restrictive or a malabsorption procedure – still goes on. What is not clear is whether they are mutually exclusive or complementary, have specific indications, or represent two different possibly successive stages of a single therapy.[27] There has generally been agreement that gastric bypass of one form or another gives better results than gastric restrictive surgery, although robust long-term data are still needed to confirm this view. There is no doubt that gastric restrictive surgery has made a comeback with the increasing use of gastric bands and the ability to insert these bands laparoscopically.

In open surgery, Jones has been making a plea for a return to the left subcostal incision claiming less wound complications.[28] All patients have a higher risk of postoperative deep vein thrombosis despite adequate prophylaxis which means extra vigilance is necessary.[29]

RESTRICTIVE PROCEDURES

Vertical banded gastroplasty (VBG)

In many institutions, open VBG (Fig. 1A) remains the operation of choice because of its simplicity and relatively good long-term results. It would appear that the best results come from a smaller pouch of 10–15 ml with a 5 cm circumference of the stoma (VBG5). Mason is probably the best exponent of the procedure and reports a re-operation rate of 0.85% per year.[30] The argument as to what is the best material for making the band is always controversial, but there is some evidence that Dacron (woven polyester) is superior to Marlex polypropylene mesh.[31] Some surgeons prefer Gortex (polytetrafluroethylene). The technique of vertical stapling is controversial because of the well-recognised late staple line failures. On comprehensively reviewing the situation, Dietel suggests that the optimal technique is still not clear.[32] Increasingly, surgeons are using 2 or 3 applications of the TA-90B in order to minimise staple line breakdown.[33] Importantly, the stoma should not be too tight and probably the vertical staple line should not be oversewn. Some surgeons divide the vertical staple to decrease staple line dehiscence, but this is not appealing to others because of the theoretically increased likelihood of gastric leak. A report from Norway, where VBG patients received 24 h pH studies before and after surgery, showed that VBG did not demonstrate anti-reflux properties as is commonly believed.[34] This was also confirmed by another study from Sweden.[35]

There have also been increasing reports of laparoscopic VBG, a technically demanding operation, with good results in experienced hands. Probably the largest experience is that of Lonroth from Sweden who has obtained excellent results comparable with published series of open VBG.[36] A compromise may be to use a hand-assisted laparoscopic technique especially to manipulate the head of the circular stapler.[37]

Gastric banding

Interest is accruing rapidly in performing gastric banding (Fig. 1A) especially in Europe and Australia. There are two main bands, a Swedish Adjustable

Silicone Band (SAGB) and an American Adjustable Silicone Gastric Band (ASGB). No formal comparisons have been made between the two bands.

The ASGB was originally placed in the patient by an open technique. Now most are being placed laparoscopically, hence the band is now called the Lap-Band. There have been 23,000 inserted world-wide with many reports of its efficacy. Probably the largest personal series is that of Belachew from Belgium who has inserted 450, most of them laparoscopically. At 6 years' follow-up,

(A) Gastric restriction

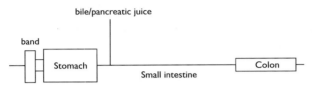

(B) Gastric bypass

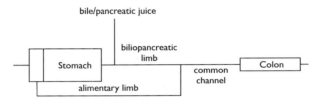

(C) Biliopancreatic diversion

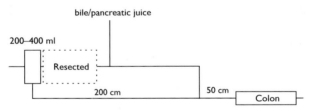

(D) Biliopancreatic diversion with duodenal switch

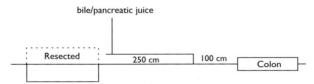

(E) Jejuno-ileal bypass (Cleator)

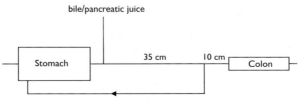

Fig. 1 Types of bariatric surgery for morbid obesity.

50–60% of excess weight has been lost although he does report a tendency to regain weight in the long-term.[38] He also emphasises the need to insert the band above the lesser sac through the bare area of the stomach in order to avoid posterior gastric prolapse. Another large series from Australia of 302 patients revealed 68.2% weight loss at 4 years although the number of patients followed up was very small.[39] As with Belachew, this author also has overcome the learning curve and modified the technique resulting in a very low complication rate with no prolapses or re-operations in his last 100 patients.

The Swedish SAGB has been widely reported by various authors. Some surgeons are having disappointing results although they are probably still optimising their technique.[40] Perhaps the leading Swedish exponent of the band technique is Forsell and colleagues who recently published a long-term follow-up of 326 patients.[41] The mean excess weight loss was 68% with an early complication rate of around 7%. Most of these were related to the learning curve of devising the optimal positioning, inflation and fixation technique. The most serious complication is migration-erosion (4.7%), which is likely to decrease with knowledge of likely causes, e.g. band over-inflation.

Although no randomised studies have been performed with these bands, either against each other or other standard procedures such as VBG or GBP, there is a general feeling amongst the bariatric community that they are worth considering in selected patients. Indeed, many surgeons now use gastric banding as their main bariatric procedure. Despite lack of good data attesting to their long-term durability, there is an increasing swing towards banding especially if they can be placed laparoscopically which reduces morbidity for the patient. Furthermore, the banding procedure is less destructive to the stomach and has the potential for complete reversibility if an effective medical cure is ever found for morbid obesity. There is also a prevalent view that since the laparoscopic banding procedure is relatively harmless then options still remain open for subsequent open operations for banding failures. However, banding has the additional expense of the prosthesis and instrumentation for its insertion. Several visits are often necessary to the radiology department to get the balloon inflated to the right diameter – usually decided by trial and error. Long-term studies of the durability of gastric bands are keenly awaited.

Gastric bypass

Many US centres for obesity surgery favour gastric bypass (GBP; Fig. 1B) in one of its forms having given up gastric restrictive procedures because of their lesser efficacy. Certainly, there is ample evidence from large series and one randomised study[42] that GBP is more effective at weight reduction than simple restrictive procedures. The evolution of its variants attests to the ingenuity of various surgeons and the quest for optimal performance. A survey of American bariatric surgeons suggested that the most preferred gastric bypass was vertical with a 20–25 ml pouch and the gastroenterostomy stoma around 12 mm diameter.[43] Additional restrictive bands or rings were not preferred. However, Fobi took exception to this survey and severely criticised it claiming that some form of additional restrictive banding is likely to be more common than the survey revealed[44] – unfortunately he had no data to substantiate this!

The length of the Roux-en-Y alimentary limb has gradually crept up from around 45 cm to as long as 200 cm for average morbidly obese patients. Sarr uses

450 cm in the superobese.[45] Freeman has reported that although weight loss increases in proportion to the length of the alimentary limb, this is at the risk of an increased incidence of diarrhoea which may not be apparent for 8–12 months after operation.[46] He has proposed the optimal length should be 180 cm except for the superobese which should be longer.

Poiries has the best follow-up data in the literature of 97% for 11–17 years with around 50% excess weight loss at 60 months.[12] Despite these good results and those of others, there is still a suspicion that there is a trend for obesity to recur to some extent. However, as cogently pointed out by Freeman, no available treatment achieves anything near this success rate.[46] Hernias and bowel obstructions tend to plague this form of surgery – something which may be reduced by those surgeons who are able to perform this laparoscopically. The literature also reminds us of the potential for vitamin and micronutrient deficiency which needs supplementation.

Critics of GBP surgery emphasise the inability to endoscope the distal stomach following staple division as a disadvantage of the procedure. There are no convincing reports in the literature suggesting that this is so.

Biliopancreatic diversion (BPD)
This procedure (Fig. 1C) is really another variant on the long limb Roux-en-Y GBP combined with a gastric resection. Introduced by Scopinario, it has found a few adherents around the world. Scopinario recently reviewed his results of 2,241 patients operated on over a 21 year period and found a mean of 75% reduction of excess weight.[47] He had an operative mortality of less than 0.5% but a 3% incidence of protein calorie malnutrition.

A variant of the BPD is to do a sleeve resection of the stomach and attach the alimentary limb to the transected first part of the duodenum (duodenal switch) which gives rise to a long biliopancreatic limb (Fig. 1D). The rationale for the duodenal switch is to reduce the parietal cell area and hence the risk of stomal ulceration. Hess reported recently his experience of 440 patients undergoing this switch procedure.[48] He claimed a 70% excess weight loss at 8 years' follow-up with minimal regain of weight and 93% of patients reporting an excellent or good result. A Spanish group has also reported their preliminary results on 60 patients with this switch procedure.[49] In their experience, it was found to be an unsafe operation with a 3.3% early mortality, a 3.57% late mortality and a 5.3% conversion rate. Although weight loss was excellent they cautioned against this technique. This is a big operation which many bariatric surgeons appear reluctant to undertake as a primary procedure.

Other procedures
Jejuno-ileal bypass (JIB) is now considered by most bariatric surgeons to be of historical interest only. However, in some situations it may still be applicable especially as a temporary procedure in superobese patients prior to converting to a another procedure. The procedure is still carried out in some centres where they claim good results by avoiding the complications attributed to the bypassed segment. An example is that of Cleator and colleagues from Canada where they implant the bypassed segment into the upper stomach in a retrograde manner (Fig. 1E).[50] They claim excellent weight loss and low morbidity. Frandson and colleagues from Denmark recently reported their follow-up of 57 patients after

JIB.[51] There was a 19% re-operation rate and 12% late mortality although none were related to the JIB. Most of the re-operations were for JIB related complications; therefore, they felt they could not recommended this operation as a routine.

Although endoscopic insertion of free floating gastric balloons are not operations they have made a recent re-appearance after a period of neglect. They went through a phase of use of the late 1980s, then disillusionment set in when they were perceived to have difficulties. A new balloon from the Bioenteric Corporation is currently being widely used and some early results look promising with 10–25 kg weight loss[52]. However, they are only a stop-gap manoeuvre and need to be part of a vigorous diet programme.

Key point 6 & 7

- More research needs to be done on the relative merits of the various surgical procedures which are available.
- Laparoscopic bariatric surgery needs careful evaluation.

REDO SURGERY

Like any redo gastric surgery, it is attended by greater morbidity and mortality and is not for the faint hearted. Nevertheless, all bariatric surgeons should have the skills to undertake this surgery. The literature has several reports of anecdotes about favourite conversions. For example, Capella favours converting a failed VBG to a GBP and gives good operative tips from his experience of 60 cases.[53] Similar good results have been reported by Gemert[54] and Sugerman.[55] Another report of 63 conversions from the US emphasises the good results and safety in experienced hands.[56]

SUGGESTED ALGORITHM

Based on the foregoing, it is difficult to give advice about which procedures to perform for the surgeon wishing to undertake this form of surgery. There is probably no one operation that is suitable for all-comers. Like so much surgery, personal preferences and training often influence the choices made. In an ideal world, all bariatric surgeons would be completely familiar with all bariatric procedures but this is rarely so. The interested surgeon should seek training from experienced colleagues, preferably those who are recognised by their peer group as having special expertise in this area. The Cancun statement adopted by the International Federation for Surgery of Obesity for credentialling bariatric surgeons is a step in the right direction, but may be hard to achieve in all countries at present until there is a trained cohort of bariatric surgeons.[57]

The author's own algorithm in shown in Figure 2. However, all patients must be taken on their own merits and guidelines should not be too slavishly adhered to, since the evidence base for them is still wanting. Patients must be

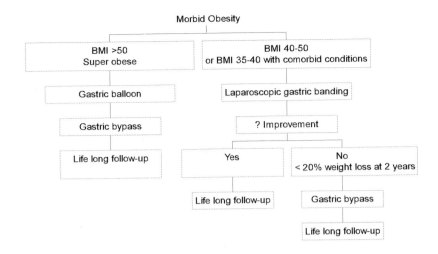

Fig. 2 Algorithm for managing morbidly obese patients suitable for surgery.

involved in the decision making. There is certainly a feeling that laparoscopic banding is a lot more minimalist for a first procedure and may be used to select patients for subsequent surgery should that prove necessary.

USEFUL INTERNET SITES

American Bariatric Surgery Society – http://www.asbs.org/
International Federation for Surgery of Obesity – http://www.obesity-online.com/ifso
International Bariatric Surgery Registry – http://surgery.uiowa.edu/nbsr/ibsrbroc.html

---

Key points for clinical practice

- .Prejudice against bariatric surgery is still rife.

- Public and health care provider awareness of the cost-effectiveness of bariatric surgery needs to be emphasised.

- The Swedish Obesity Subjects study will have an enormous impact on the role of bariatric surgery when the study is fully reported.

- Bariatric surgery should only be carried out within the context of an obesity team.

- Good long-term audit of surgical results needs to be carried out.

- More research needs to be done on the relative merits of the various surgical procedures which are available.

- Laparoscopic bariatric surgery needs careful evaluation.

References

1. Maddi S R, Khoshaba D M, Persico M et al. Psychological correlates of psychopathology in a national sample of the morbidly obese. Obes Surg 1997; 7: 397–404.
2. National Institutes of Health Consensus statement – Gastrointestinal surgery for severe obesity. Nutrition 1996; 12: 397–402.
3. Scottish Intercollegiate Guidelines Network. Obesity in Scotland: Integrating Prevention with Health Management. Scottish Intercollegiate Guidelines Network. November 1996.
4. Wright P D. The current status of bariatric surgery in the UK. Obes Surg; 1998: 8: 364–365.
5. Cowan G S M. What do patients, families and society expect from the bariatric surgeon? Obes Surg 1998; 8: 77–85.
6. Powers P S, Rosemurgy A, Boyd F et al. Outcome of gastric restriction procedures: weight, psychiatric diagnoses and satisfaction. Obes Surg 1997; 7: 471–477.
7. Choi Y, Frizzi J, Foley A et al. Patient satisfaction and results of vertical banded gastroplasty and gastric bypass. Obes Surg 1999; 9: 33–35.
8. Isacsson A, Frederiksen S G, Nilsson P et al. Quality of life after gastroplasty is normal: a controlled study. Eur J Surg 1997; 163: 181–186.
9. Wolf A M, Beisiegel U, Kortner B et al. Does gastric restriction surgery reduce the risks of metabolic diseases? Obes Surg 1998; 8: 9–13.
10. King R F G J, Dachtler J, Johnston D et al. A simple gastric restrictive procedure cures diabetes and reverses dyslipidaemia in obese patients. Br J Surg 1999; 86 (Suppl. 1): 93.
11. Dachtler J, Johnston D, King R F G J et al. The treatment of hypercholesterolaemia by partial ileal resection. Br J Surg 1999; 86 (Suppl. 1); 74–75.
12. Pories W J, Swanson M S, MacDonald K G, Long S B, Mavis P G, Brown B M. Who would have thought it? An operation proves to be the most effective therapy for adult-onset diabetes mellitus. Ann Surg 1995; 222: 339–352.
13. Gahtan V, Goode S E, Kurto H Z et al. Body composition and source of weight loss after bariatric surgery. Obes Surg 1997; 7: 184–188.
14. Karason K, Wallentin I, Larsson B et al. Effect of obesity and weight loss on cardiac function and valvular performance. Obes Res 1998; 6: 422–429.
15. Karlsson J, Sjostrom L, Sullivan M. Swedish obese subjects (SOS) – an intervention study of obesity. Int J Obes Relat Metab Disord 1998; 22: 113–126.
16. Ghasssemian A J, MacDonald K G, Cunningham P G et al. The workup for bariatric surgery does not require a routine upper gastrointestinal series. Obes Surg 1997; 7: 16–18.
17. Verset D, HouBen J J, Gay F et al. The place of upper gastrointestinal tract endoscopy before and after vertical banded gastroplasty for morbid obesity. Dig Dis Sci 1997; 42: 2333–2337.
18. Pelosi P, Croci M, Ravagnan I et al. The effects of body mass on lung volumes, respiratory mechanics, and gas exchange during general anesthesia. Anesth Analg 1998; 87: 654–660.
19. Dumont L, Mattys M, Mardirosoff C et al. Changes in pulmonary mechanics during laparoscopic gastroplasty in morbidly obese patients. Acta Anaesth Scand 1997; 41: 408–413.
20. Dumont L, Mattys M, Mardirosoff C et al. Hemodynamic changes during laparoscopic gastroplasty in morbidly obese patients. Obes Surg 1997; 7: 326–331.
21. Bloomston M, Zervos E E, campus M A et al. Outcome following bariatric surgery in super versus morbidly obese patients: does weight matter? Obes Surg 1997; 7: 414–419.
22. Deitel M. Pregnancy after bariatric surgery. Obes Surg 1998; 8: 465–466.
23. Bianco A T, Scott W S, Davis Y et al. Pregnancy outcome and weight gain recommendations for the morbidly obese woman. Obstet Gynecol 1998; 91: 97–102.
24. Hsu L K G, Benotti P N, Dwyer J et al. Nonsurgical factors that influence the outcome of bariatric surgery: a review. Pyschosom Med 1998; 60: 338–346.
25. Alvarez-Cordero R. World progress in surgery: treatment of clinically severe obesity, a public health problem. World J Surg 1998; 22: 905–906.
26. Mason E E, Tang S, Renquist K E et al. A decade of change in obesity surgery. Obes Surg 1997; 7: 189–197.
27. Forestieri P, De Luca M, Formato A et al. Restrictive versus malabsorption procedures: criteria for patient selection. Obes Surg 1999; 9: 48–50.
28. Jones K B. The left subcostal incision revisited. Obes Surg 1998; 8: 225–228.
29. Eriksson S, Backman L, Ljungstrom K. The incidence of clinical postoperative thrombosis

after gastric surgery for obesity during 16 years. Obes Surg 1997; 7: 332–335.

30. Mason E E. Change in obesity surgery. Obes Surg 1997; 7: 373

31. van Gemert W G, Greve J W M, Soeters P B. Long-term results of vertical banded gastroplasty: Marlex versus Dacron banding. Obes Surg 1997; 7: 128–135.

32. Deitel M. Staple disruption in VBG. Obes Surg 1997; 7: 139–141.

33. Fobi M A L. Rediscovering the wheel in obesity surgery. Obes Surg 1997; 7: 370–372.

34. Ovrebo K K, Hatlebakk J G, Viste A et al. Gastroesophageal reflux in morbidly obese patients treated with gastric banding or veryical banded gastroplasty. Ann Surg 1998; 228: 51–58.

35. Naslund E, Granstrom L, Melcher A et al. Gastro-oesophageal reflux before and after vertical banded gastroplasty in the treatment of obesity. Eur J Surg 1996; 162: 303–306.

36. Lonroth H, Dalenbeck J. Other laparoscopic bariatric procedures. World J Surg 1998; 22: 964–968.

37. Watson D I, Game P A. Hand-assisted laparoscopic vertical banded gastroplasty. Surg Endosc 1997; 11: 1218–1220

38. Belachew M, Legrand M, Vincent V et al. Laparoscopic adjustable gastric banding. World J Surg 1998; 22: 955–963.

39. O'Brien P E, Brown W A, Smith P J et al. Prospective study of a laparoscopically placed, adjustable gastric band in the treatment of morbid obesity. Br J Surg 1999; 85: 113–118.

40. Westling A, Bjurling K, Ohrvall M et al. Silicone-adjustable gastric banding: disappointing results. Obes Surg 1998; 8: 467–474.

41. Forsell P, Hallerback B, Glise H et al. Complications following Swedish adjustable gastric banding: a long-trem follow-up. Obes Surg 1999; 9: 11–16.

42. Sugerman H J, Starkey J V, Birkenhauer R. A randomised prospective trial of gastric bypass versus vertical banded gastroplasty for morbid obesity and their effects on sweets versus non-sweets eaters. Ann Surg 1987; 205: 613–622.

43. Talieh J, Kirgan D, Fisher BL. Gastric bypass for morbid obesity: a standard surgical technique by consensus. Obes Surg 1997; 7: 198–202.

44. Fobi M A L. Gastric bypass: standard surgical technique. Obes Surg 1997; 7: 518–520.

45. Sarr M G, Felty C L, Hilmer D M et al. Technical and practical considerations involved in operations on patients weighing more than 270 kg. Arch Surg 1995; 130: 102–105.

46. Freeman J B, Kotlarewsky M, Phoenix C. Weight loss after extended gastric bypass. Obes Surg 1997; 7: 337–344.

47. Scopinario N, Adami GF, Marinari G M et al. Biliopancreatic diversion. World J Surg 1998; 22: 936–946.

48. Hess D S, Hess D W. Biliopancreatic diversion with a duodenal switch. Obes Surg 1998; 8: 267–282.

49. Baltasar A, del Rio J, Escriva C et al. Preliminary results of the duodenal switch. Obes Surg 1997; 7: 500–504.

50. Cleator I G M, Gourlay R H. Ileogastrostomy for morbid obesity. Can J Surg 1988; 31: 114–116.

51. Frandsen J, Pedersen S B, Richelsen B. Long term follow up of patients who underwent jejunoileal bypass for morbid obesity. Eur J Surg 1998; 164: 281–286.

52. Galloro G, DePalma G D, Catanzanzano C et al. Preliminary endoscopic technical report of a new silicone intragastric balloon in the treatment of morbid obesity. Obes Surg 1999; 9: 68–71.

53. Capella R F, Capella J F. Converting vertical banded gastroplasty to a lesser curvature gastric bypass: technical considerations. Obes Surg 1998; 8: 218–224.

54. Van Gemert W G, van Wersch M M, Greve J W M et al. Revisional surgery after failed vertical banded gastroplasty: restoration of vertical banded gastroplasty or conversion to gastric bypass. Obes Surg 1998; 8: 21–28.

55. Sugerman H J, Kellum J M, DeMaria E J et al. Conversion of failed or complicated veryical banded gastroplasty to gastric bypass in morbid obesity. Am J Surg 1996; 171: 263–269.

56. Benotti P N, Forse R A. Safety and long-term efficacy of revisional surgery in severe obesity. Am J Surg 1996; 172: 232–235.

57. Cowan G S M. The Cancun IFSO statement on bariatric surgeon qualifications. Obes Surg 1998; 8: 86

Mohammad R. S. Keshtgar Peter J. Ell

Sentinel lymph node biopsy in breast carcinoma

The status of the axilla in patients with breast cancer and its impact on management remain the subject of intense debate. The histological examination of axillary lymph nodes remains the most reliable technique to determine the nodal status in breast carcinoma but the need for and extent of axillary lymph node dissection (ALND) is controversial. ALND has remained an integral part of breast cancer management for over a century, despite a tendency towards a more conservative approach to breast surgery. Evidence of the spread of cancer to the axilla is still considered the single most important prognostic indicator in breast cancer patients. Whilst the value of ALND in loco-regional control is beyond dispute, it does not seem to have a significant effect on long-term survival.

Axillary staging in breast cancer can help in rational decision making about adjuvant systemic therapy but such decisions can also be made without reference to lymph nodal status. Currently, adjuvant systemic therapy in the form of cytotoxic chemotherapy or hormonal therapy alone or in combination is recommended for most invasive breast cancers. The recent world overview of the Early Breast Cancer Trialists' Collaborative Group[1] on adjuvant polychemotherapy indicates that the proportional risk reduction for recurrence and mortality appears to be the same for node negative and node positive breast cancer patients, although in terms of a 10 year survival span the absolute benefit is 7% for those with node negative disease and 11% for those with node positive disease.

Recent epidemiological studies indicate that breast cancers are smaller in size at presentation and have less likelihood of lymph node involvement than

Mr Mohammad R.S. Keshtgar BSc MB BS FRCSI FRCS(Gen), Clinical Lecturer/Surgical Oncologist, Academic Department of Surgery and Institute of Nuclear Medicine, Royal Free and University College Medical School, University College London, Mortimer Street, London W1N 8AA, UK (correspondence)

Prof. Peter J. Ell MD PD MSc FRCR FRCP, Professor and Head of Institute of Nuclear Medicine, Royal Free and University College Medical School, University College London, Mortimer Street, London W1N 8AA, UK

Table 1 The results of four studies with a total number of 4,937 patients analysed to determine the frequency of lymph node positivity according to the tumour size.[4]

Author	Group size	T1a (<0.5 cm)	T1b (0.5–1.0 cm)	T1c (1.0–2.0 cm)	T2 (2.0–5.0 cm)
Silverstein	1031	3	17	32	44
McGee	3077	12	23	33	54
Giuliano	259	10	13	30	–
Cady	570	–	17	31	44
Weighted average	4937	7%	19%	32%	51%

in the past. This could be as a result of widespread use of mammographic screening and the increase in patients' awareness.[2,3] In a study performed by Silverstein et al,[2] in 1031 patients with breast carcinoma – looking at axillary nodal involvement, disease-free survival and breast cancer specific survival in six breast cancer subgroups (Tis [DCIS], T1a, T1b, T1c, T2 and T3) – it was noted that nodal involvement in DCIS was 0%; T1a 3%; T1b 17%; T1c 32%; T2 44%; T3 60%. The authors suggest routine ALND should no longer be performed in patients with T1a (< 0.5 cm) breast carcinoma, as only 3% are likely to have axillary nodes involved with metastatic carcinoma. Table 1 summarises the results of four studies with a total number of 4,937 patients analysed to determine the frequency of lymph node positivity according to the tumour size.[4]

Up to 70% of patients with T1/T2 tumours fail to show any evidence of nodal involvement after ALND[5] and more than 50% of these node negative patients will develop a complication of the operation.[3,6] These include postoperative pain, seroma formation, limitation of shoulder movements, parasthesia and numbness of the upper arm, inadvertent damage to neurovascular structures and the distressing complication of lymphoedema. Moreover, hospital stay is prolonged with cost implications. It is ironic that the extent, morbidity and cost of a staging procedure (ALND) is greater than the surgical treatment of the primary tumour. It is hence difficult to justify performing ALND routinely in all breast cancer patients.

SENTINEL NODE CONCEPT

The concept of the sentinel lymph node (SLN) and biopsy of this node is based on the hypothesis that lymph flow is orderly and predictable and tumour cells disseminate sequentially. The sentinel node is the first node encountered by tumour cells and its histological status predicts distant lymph basin status (Table 2).

The SLN is defined as the lymph node(s) which is in a direct drainage pathway from the primary tumour. It is at the highest risk of harbouring metastatic deposits. A second echelon node receives lymph from the SLN (first echelon node).

In 1891, Halsted described his concept of centrifugal spread of breast cancer,[7] regarding the lymphatic route as the most significant mechanism of

Table 2 Sentinel lymph node concept. The sentinel node is the first node encountered by tumour cells and its histological status predicts distant lymph basin status

- Lymph flow is orderly and predictable
- Tumour cells disseminate sequentially
- The Sentinel lymph node is the first node that meets tumour cells
- Sentinel lymph node histological status predicts distant basin status
- Disease presents earlier and basin involvement is less frequent, therefore surgery can be targeted to the appropriate population

tumour dissemination in breast cancer. He also proposed that the lymphatic spread of the tumour is orderly and predictable, and that the lymph nodes were the source of distant metastasis (Fig. 1).

In 1977, Cabanas[8] was the first person to introduce the sentinel node biopsy as a staging procedure in penile carcinoma by directly injecting contrast medium into the dorsal lymphatics of the penis in patients with penile carcinoma. The first visualised lymph node was designated the sentinel lymph node. In 1992, Morton and co-workers[9] applied this concept to malignant melanoma using blue dye. In 1993, Alex and associates[10] injected a radio-pharmaceutical (^{99m}Tc-sulphur colloid) and introduced the technique of gamma probe guided surgery. Following the success of the sentinel node concept in melanoma, it was applied to breast cancer.[11]

The potential advantages of SLN detection and biopsy are:

1. *It is a minimally invasive technique which can reduce morbidity and cost.[12]*

2. *By identifying one or two lymph nodes that are most likely to be involved with metastatic deposit, pathologists can perform a more detailed histological analysis.*

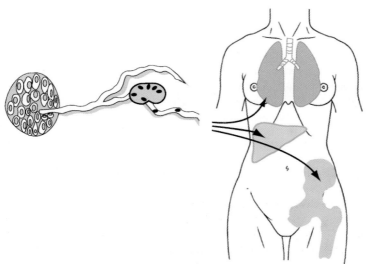

Fig. 1 A representation of the concept of 'orderly metastatic spread' of breast cancer.

This will increase the detection rate of micrometastatic disease. A SLN biopsy may become more sensitive than ALND in diagnosing axillary nodal metastasis.

3. *Nodal metastasis outside the axilla can be detected.*

4. *This approach may obviate the need for routine ALND in all breast cancer patients without compromising staging information, local control or long-term survival.*

It is relevant here to emphasise that the SLN biopsy is a diagnostic test and that before it is accepted for routine clinical use, its accuracy has to be established. The critical issue is the false negative rate. Presently ALND is associated with a false negative rate of up to 3%.[13,14] It is difficult to determine what is an acceptable false negative rate.[15] 'At what stage does the benefit of a less invasive staging investigation overweigh the risk of a false negative result?'[16]

At present there is no standardised technique for performing the SLN biopsy and there is variation in practice in almost every aspect of this procedure. These include patient selection, particle size of the radiopharmaceuticals, radiation detectors, injection technique, imaging technique, detection technique and the gathering of pathological evidence from the specimen.[17] Despite this variation, the overall results are encouraging. A combined analysis of 1,385 patients with breast carcinoma by McMasters et al[16] leads to an overall sensitivity of 94% and 100% specificity with a false negative rate of 6.2%, when the sentinel node technique was performed in patients who also had ALND. The overall accuracy is 98% with a positive predictive value of 100% and a negative predictive value of 97% (Table 3).

PATIENT SELECTION

The criteria for patient selection for SLN biopsy at our institution are as follows.

ELIGIBILITY CRITERIA

All patients with palpable or non-palpable carcinoma of the breast (T1, T2) on triple assessment, i.e. clinical examination, imaging (mammogram and ultrasound) and tissue diagnosis (cytology, Tru-cut biopsy), where surgical treatment would involve removal of the primary tumour and axillary lymph node dissection.

EXCLUSION CRITERIA

1. Patients with clinically involved axilla.

2. Pregnant and lactating women.

3. Patients with multifocal/multicentric carcinomas of the breast.

4. Patients with previous breast surgery on the same side.

Table 3 A combined analysis of SLN biopsy with concomitant ALND in patients with carcinoma breast, from McMasters et al [16]

No. of patients with SLN identified (%)	1385
Technique	All techniques
Sensitivity (%)	94
Specificity (%)	100
Positive predictive value (%)	100
Negative predictive value (%)	97
Overall accuracy (%)	98
SLN only positive node (%)	48
False negative rate (%)	6.2

It is important to exclude patients with a clinically involved axillary lymph node. This is one of the potential pitfalls in the sentinel node localization and can lead to a false negative result.[18] This is likely to be due to a change in the lymphatic flow as a result of replacement of the sentinel node with metastatic carcinoma. The colloid bypasses the sentinel node and moves on to a non-sentinel lymph node. Previous breast surgery should not be regarded as an absolute contra-indication for sentinel node biopsy. It seems that the success rate of sentinel node localisation is lower in patients with previous breast surgery,[19] although the false negative rate is not affected.[18] Multifocal tumours are likely to involve more than one lymphatic trunk from the mammary gland to the axillary nodes which may give rise to a false negative result.[20,21]

TECHNETIUM-99m LABELLED COLLOID PARTICLES

The tracers used for lymphoscintigraphy are colloidal albumin labelled with technetium-99m with a physical half-life of 6 h and an imaging energy of 140 keV. The colloidal particles enter the lymphatics through patent junctions between endothelial cells and are carried to the first draining lymph node. These particles are taken up by the reticuloendothelial system, mainly

---

Key point 1

- The sentinel node concept is validated in breast carcinoma.

Key point 2

- Patients with a clinically involved axilla or a multifocal breast cancer should be excluded from the sentinel node biopsy. There is a higher incidence of false negative rate associated with these conditions.

macrophages, giving rise to increased focal radioactivity within the lymph node. This allows its detection during imaging as a hot spot and at operation using a gamma-detection probe. It must be emphasised that these radioactive particles find the first draining lymph node(s) irrespective of whether they are involved with carcinoma or not; in other words, they are lymph-node-seeking-agents and not tumour-seeking-agents.[22]

It seems that the particle size plays an important role in successful localisation of the SLN. There is a need to identify an ideal colloid for sentinel lymph node visualisation, which is clearly different from a particulate tracer which is optimised for the visualisation of all lymph nodes. The exact range of particle sizes should be known, the product should be stable on storage, that it should be labelled with technetium-99m and, for the purpose of sentinel lymph node detection, it should contain particles of an average size of the order of 80–200 nm.[17] Uren et al present an opposing view and firmly believe that only small size tracer with a range of 5–50 nm will clearly succeed in mapping of the SLN.

INJECTION TECHNIQUES

There are significant variations in the administration technique of the radiopharmaceutical. These vary from a single subdermal injection to multiple peritumoral injections and even intra-tumoral injection (Fig. 2). The other variables include the injection volume and dosage. The injection can be administered the day before operation or on the same day according to the agreed protocol.

Subdermal injection

On the day preceding operation, a single dose of 10–15 MBq of [^{99m}Tc]-labelled Nanocoll in a volume of 0.2 ml is injected subdermally at the tumour site (Fig. 3), using a 25 G needle. This technique is based on the fact that the breast is developmentally derived from the ectoderm and the dermal and parenchymal lymphatics of breast meet at the sub-areolar lymphatic plexus[23] and from here one to two main lymphatic trunks drain towards the axilla. Sappey's illustration of one or two large collecting lymph trunks originating from the subareolar lymphatic plexus has been confirmed by other investigators using direct lymphangiographic techniques.[24] Borgstein and co-workers[25] confirmed the hypothesis that the lymphatics of the overlying skin drain to the same axillary sentinel node as the underlying glandular breast tissue. We have recently reported a new technique for the delivery of the radiopharmaceutical using a needle-free injection system[26] with encouraging results. The advantage of this technique is that the administration of the radionuclide is virtually pain-free which makes the procedure more acceptable to the patient.

Peri-tumour injection

This technique is commonly practised. The radiocolloid is injected around the tumour into the breast parenchyma. With this technique, removal of the tracer and the dye is slower due to a relatively scantier lymphatic supply of the breast parenchyma.[27] In this setting, dynamic imaging is less useful since one is less likely to see the lymphatic tract. Imaging is commonly performed 1–2 h after the injection is administered. A larger injection volume is given with this technique. The injection is usually given at four sites: superior, inferior, medial and lateral to the tumour.

LYMPHOSCINTIGRAPHY

This is usually performed a day before operation. The purpose of this procedure is to find the location and number of the SLN pre-operatively. It also helps to

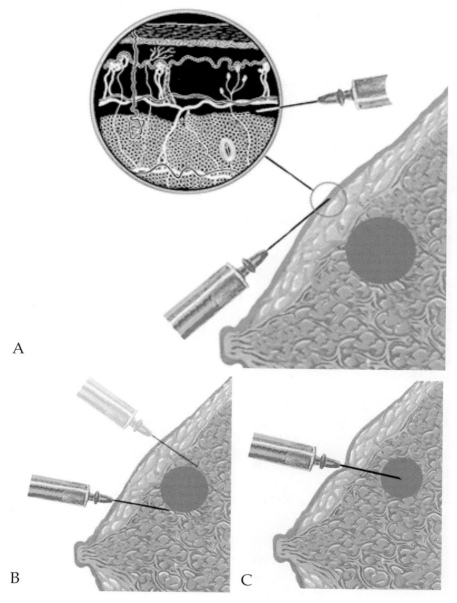

A

B

C

Fig. 2 Possible route for administration of tracer for sentinel node detection.
(**A**) Subdermal injection. (**B**) Peri-tumour injection. (**C**) Intra-tumour injection.[17]

differentiate the SLN from second and third echelon nodes and offers the surgeon a useful road map. Once the radiopharmaceutical is administered, the drainage and retention of the particles by the lymphatic system can be

Key point 3

- There is no standard technique for administration of radionuclide. Subdermal injection is a fast and reliable technique with a good success rate for sentinel node localisation. Peri-tumour injection is a commonly practised procedure. The flow of tracer is slower and a larger volume of the injectate at multiple sites is required for this technique to be successful.

Key point 4

- It is important to observe good radiation safety procedures during administration of radiocolloid.

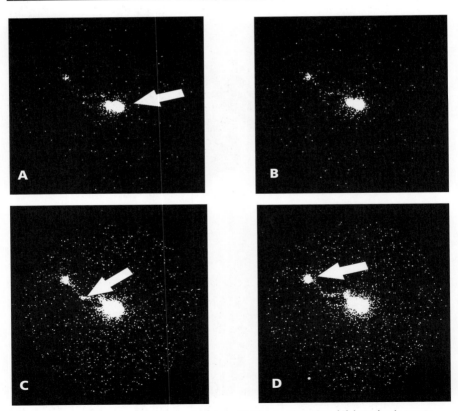

Fig. 3 Dynamic imaging sequence showing: (**A,B**) injection site; (**C**) lymphatic tract; and (**D**) the sentinel lymph node.

investigated accurately. Imaging devices (such as the conventional Anger gamma camera) are ideally suited to record this.[17] Dynamic imaging (Fig. 3), although not an essential part of breast lymphoscintigraphy, will give a rapid indication of the progress of the radiocolloid from the administered site, and the lymphatic tract(s) is usually visible. It will also allow for an early warning, should the tracer fail to migrate. Static imaging is performed in two views, the anterior and the lateral projection. To outline the patient's body profile during imaging, a ^{57}Co flood source is used beneath the patient and a transmission image is obtained (Fig. 4).

THE SURGICAL TECHNIQUE

The surgical approach to the intra-operative detection of a sentinel node varies significantly. It may range from blue dye lymphatic mapping alone to probe guided surgery alone or in combination with blue dye technique.

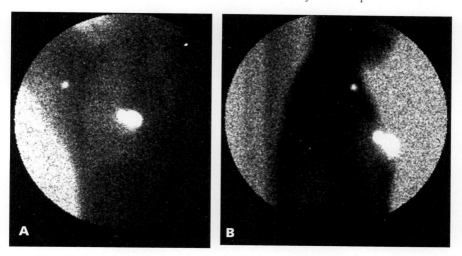

Fig. 4 Static imaging with ^{57}Co flood source: **(A)** anterior-oblique view; **(B)** lateral view.

BLUE DYE LYMPHATIC MAPPING

With intraparenchymal injection of the blue dye alone, the success rate for identification of the SLN varies between 65–93%.[28,29] Giuliano et al[30] performed lymphatic mapping by using isosulfan blue vital dye which was injected in a peritumoural fashion into the breast parenchyma in 174 patients with a success rate of 65% and sensitivity of 75%, although the success rate has improved with experience in recent reports. This technique can be tedious and a significant training element is necessary.[31] The extent of the dissection and disruption of lymphatic channels is higher as compared to probe guided surgery since the success of this technique depends on tracing the blue lymphatic ducts that lead to the SLN. Moreover, localisation of sentinel nodes in lymphatic basins other than the axillary basin is not possible.[32] Timing of

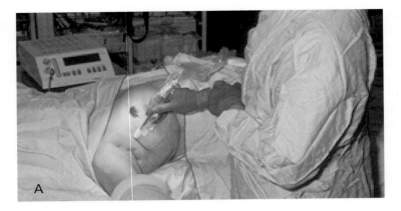

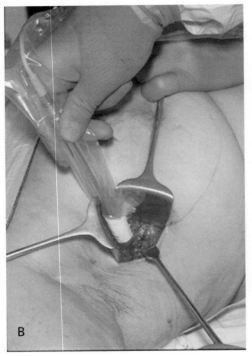

Fig. 5 (**A**) Determination of the sentinel lymph node site before incision, the gamma probe display unit faces the surgeon. Arrow points to the site of the blue dye injection. (**B**) Sentinel lymph node localised with the gamma probe. Additional visual assistance from the blue dye is complementary.

injection of blue dye is a crucial factor for the success of the procedure. Patients should be warned about blue discoloration of urine and persistence of a blue stain in the breast.

PROBE GUIDED SURGERY

The success rate for operation guided by a gamma detection probe is superior to blue dye mapping alone.[18–20] In a pilot study performed by Krag and associates,[11] the technique of probe-guided localization of radiolabelled sentinel lymph node was introduced after its initial success in staging melanoma patients. The success rate of this technique was 82% with a predictive accuracy of 100%. In a study performed by Albertini and associates,[19] combining the blue dye and probe-guided operation in 62 patients, a success rate of 92% was reported with 100% accuracy in predicting axillary node status. Addition of gamma detection probe increased the success rate from 73% to 92%, as in 12 patients blue dye did not appear in the lymph nodes, whilst focal increased activity was detected by the gamma probe. They concluded that blue dye lymphatic mapping and probe-guided sentinel node localisation are complementary. Other investigators share this view[18,20] and argue that the incidence of false negative results is reduced when the techniques are combined. This may also accelerate the learning curve of each method used in isolation.

We have adopted a policy of pre-operative lymphoscintigraphy and the combination of blue dye lymphatic mapping and probe-guided operation for intra-operative localisation of the sentinel lymph node. It has been our experience that additional information from pre-operative lymphoscintigraphy is very helpful in accurate localisation of the SLN.

The steps involved at operation are summarised below.

Determination of the site of incision

The location of the sentinel node before the incision can be verified by a gamma detecting probe (Fig. 5A). This helps the surgeon to decide where to place the incision.

Establishment of the 'line-of-sight'

This is one of the important advantages of probe guided surgery,[11] as it gives the surgeon a sense of direction. In this way the dissection is not blind and the surgeon determines the shortest route to the sentinel node by changing the angle of the probe tip. As a result, tissue disruption is minimal.

Excision of the sentinel node

After the sentinel node is localised by the probe, additional visual assistance from the blue dye is complementary. The radioactivity of the node is recorded by the probe as 'in vivo counts/s' (Fig. 5B). The radioactive node is excised and the 'ex-vivo' count is measured. The sentinel node is labelled separately and sent fresh to the laboratory for further analysis.

Verification of sentinel node excision

It is very important to confirm the complete removal of the radioactive nodes. This is achieved by re-applying the probe in to the wound and a careful measurement of the residual activity.

Completion lymphadenectomy

At present, after the sentinel node is excised, the standard axillary node dissection is performed, as we are validating the predictive value of sentinel node biopsy in determining the status of the axillary lymphatic basin. It is hoped that SLN biopsy will in future permit selective axillary dissection.

Key points 5–7

- The gamma detection probe enables the surgeon to determine the site of incision by finding the area of maximum activity. One of the greatest advantages of probe guided surgery is that complete sentinel node excision can be verified by re-applying the probe in to the wound and checking the background activity.

- Combination of the pre-operative lymphoscintigraphy, probe guided operation and blue dye technique is associated with a higher detection rate, lower false negative rate and a shorter learning period.

- There is a definite learning curve with the surgical technique; the success of the technique is operator dependent. Training and a an interactive multidisciplinary team approach are key for quality data.

PITFALLS OF SENTINEL NODE BIOPSY IN BREAST CANCER

The technique of sentinel node biopsy has recognised problems, outlined below.

REDUCED FUNCTIONAL CAPACITY OF THE SENTINEL NODE

Extensive infiltration by metastatic carcinoma

Preservation of the functional capacity of the lymph node for nodal uptake of the radioactive colloid is essential for successful localisation.[31] Nodal uptake is progressively reduced if there is excessive infiltration with metastatic carcinoma.

Excessive infiltration of the lymph node can lead to directional flow changes of lymph, leading to a 'skip phenomenon' whereby the SLN is by-passed and the radionuclide is taken up by a non-sentinel lymph node. This can cause a false negative SLN biopsy.

Fatty degeneration of the sentinel node

The other reason for reduced functional capacity of lymph node is fatty degeneration of the axillary lymph nodes. We have observed this condition in elderly patients. Tracer uptake by the lymph node is reduced, which in turn makes the probe localisation difficult.

UPPER OUTER QUADRANT LESIONS

Tumour in the upper outer quadrant can pose some difficulty during gamma probe localisation. This is due to the close proximity of the injection site to the sentinel lymph node leading to the 'shine through phenomenon'.[12] We recommend retraction of breast downward and medially during imaging and use of a collimator during probe guided surgery to overcome this problem.

PRACTICAL IMPLICATIONS

In light of information acquired to date, we propose the following approach to SLN biopsy in breast cancer.

AXILLARY MANAGEMENT IN DCIS, SMALL BREAST CANCER AND SPECIAL HISTOLOGICAL TYPE CARCINOMA

It can be argued that patients with extensive DCIS, primary breast cancers less than 0.5 cm (T1a) and also patients with specific histological type cancers (e.g. tubular, papillary and colloid), should undergo excision of the primary tumour and SLN biopsy only. If the SLN is involved, they should be offered ALND.

AXILLARY MANAGEMENT IN T1 AND T2 BREAST CANCER

This novel and promising technique should still be regarded as a research tool and, at present, SLN biopsy must be performed in a clinical trial setting. We have to await the results of ongoing randomised trials before adopting this procedure for routine management of patients with breast carcinoma.

Key point 8

- Sentinel lymph node biopsy must be performed in a trial setting. We need to await the results of ongoing randomised trials, before adopting this technique for routine use in clinical practice.

SUMMARY

The sentinel node concept is validated at least in malignant melanoma and breast carcinoma. Its success relies on proper patient selection, standardisation of various aspects of the technique and an interactive multidisciplinary team of surgeons, nuclear medicine physicians, physicists and pathologists.[33] There is a learning period associated with the technique. The results in breast cancer are encouraging but at present this procedure must be performed in a clinical trial setting.

Key points for clinical practice

- The sentinel node concept is validated in breast carcinoma.

- Patients with a clinically involved axilla or a multifocal breast cancer should be excluded from the sentinel node biopsy. There is a higher incidence of false negative rate associated with these conditions.

Key points for clinical practice (continued)

- There is no standard technique for administration of radionuclide. Subdermal injection is a fast and reliable technique with a good success rate for sentinel node localisation. Peritumour injection is a commonly practised procedure. The flow of tracer is slower and a larger volume of the injectate at multiple sites is required for this technique to be successful.

- It is important to observe good radiation safety procedures during administration of radiocolloid.

- The gamma detection probe enables the surgeon to determine the site of incision by finding the area of maximum activity. One of the greatest advantages of probe guided surgery is that complete sentinel node excision can be verified by re-applying the probe in to the wound and checking the background activity.

- Combination of the pre-operative lymphoscintigraphy, probe guided operation and blue dye technique is associated with a higher detection rate, lower false negative rate and a shorter learning period.

- There is a definite learning curve with the surgical technique and the success of the technique is operator dependent. Training and a good multidisciplinary team approach are key for success of the technique.

- SLN biopsy must be performed in a trial setting. We need to await the results of ongoing randomised trials, before adopting this technique for routine use in clinical practice.

References

1. Early Breast Cancer Trialists' Collaborative Group. Polychemotherapy for early breast cancer: an overview of the randomised trials. Lancet 1998; 352: 930–942.
2. Silverstein M J, Gierson E D, Waisman J R, Senofsky G M, Golburn W J, Gamagani P. Axillary lymph node dissection for T1a breast carcinoma. Cancer 1994; 73: 664–667.
3. Linn P P, Alison D C, Wainstock J et al. Impact of axillary lymph node dissection on the therapy of breast cancer patients. J Clin Oncol 1993; 11: 1536–1544.
4. Pijpers R. Sentinel node imaging and detection in melanoma and breast cancer. Acad Pröfscrift (Thesis) 1999; 16.
5. Pijpers R, Meijer S, Hoekstra O S et al. Impact of lymphoscintigraphy on sentinel node identification with technetium-99m-colloidal albumin in breast cancer. J Nucl Med 1997; 38: 366–368.
6. Tobin M B, Lacey H J, Meyer L, Mortimer P S. The psychological morbidity of breast cancer-related arm swelling. Cancer 1993; 72: 3248–3252.
7. Halsted W S. The results of operations for the cure of the cancer of breast performed at the Johns Hopkins Hospital from June 1889 to January 1894. Arch Surg 1894; 20: 497.
8. Cabanas R. An approach for the treatment of penile carcinoma. Cancer 1977; 39: 456–466.
9. Morton D L, Wen D R, Wong J H et al. Technical details of intraoperative lymphatic mapping for early stage melanoma. Arch Surg 1992; 127: 392–399.
10. Alex J C, Krag D N. Gamma-probe guided localization of lymph nodes. Surg Oncol 1993; 2: 2137–2143.
11. Krag D N, Weaver D L, Alex J C, Fairbank J T. Surgical resection and radiolocalization of the sentinel lymph node in breast cancer using a gamma probe. Surg Oncol 1993; 2: 335–340.

12. Keshtgar M R S, Waddington W A, Lakhani S R, Ell P J. The Sentinel Node in Surgical Oncology. Heidelberg: Springer, 1999; 1–13, 49–59, 79–89.

13. Rosen P P, Lesser M I, Kinne D W et al. Discontinuous or 'skip' metastases in breast carcinoma: analysis of 1228 axillary dissections. Ann Surg 1983; 197: 276–283.

14. Van Lancker M, Goor C, Sacre R et al. Patterns of axillary lymph node metastasis in breast cancer. Am J Clin Oncol 1995; 18: 267–272.

15. Ell P J, Keshtgar M R S. The sentinel node and lymphoscintigraphy in breast cancer. Nucl Med Commun 1999; 20: 303–305.

16. McMasters K M, Giuliano A E, Ross M I et al. Sentinel-lymph-node biopsy for breast cancer – not yet the standard of care. N Engl J Med 1998; 339: 990–995.

17. Keshtgar M R S, Ell P J. Sentinel lymph node detection and imaging. Eur J Nucl Med 999; 26: 57–67.

18. Borgstein P J, Pijpers R, Comans E F, van Diest P J, Boom R P, Meijer S. Sentinel lymph node biopsy in breast cancer: guidelines and pitfalls of lymphoscintigraphy and gamma probe detection. J Am Coll Surg 1998; 186: 275–283.

19. Albertini J J, Lyman G H, Cox C et al. Lymphatic mapping and sentinel node biopsy in the patient with breast cancer. JAMA 1996; 276: 1818–1822.

20. Veronesi U, Paganelli G, Galimberti V et al. Lancet 1997; 349: 1864–1867.

21. Veronesi U, Zurrida S, Galimberti V. Consequences of sentinel node in clinical decision making in breast cancer and prospects for future studies. Eur J Surg Oncol 1998; 24: 93–95.

22. Nieweg O E, Jansen L, Valdes Olmos R A et al. Lymphatic mapping and sentinel lymph node biopsy in breast cancer. Eur J Nucl Med 1999; 26: S11–S16.

23. Grant R N, Tabah E J, Adair F E. The surgical significance of the subareolar plexus in cancer of the breast. Surgery 1959; 33: 71–78.

24. Kett K, Varga G, Lukacs L. Direct lymphography of the breast. Lymphology 1970; 1: 3–12.

25. Borgsein P J, Meijer S, Pijpers R. Intradermal blue dye to identify sentinel lymph-node in breast cancer. Lancet 1997; 349: 1668–1669.

26. Keshtgar M R S, Barker S G E, Ell P J. Needle-free vehicle for administration of radionuclide for sentinel node biopsy. Lancet 1999; 353: 1410–1411.

27. Gulec S A, Moffat F L, Carroll R G et al. Sentinel lymph node localization in early breast cancer. J Nucl Med 1998; 39: 1388–1393.

28. Giuliano A E, Kirgan D M, Guenther J M, Morton D L. Lymphatic mapping and sentinel lymphadenectomy for breast cancer. Ann Surg 1994; 220: 391–398.

29. Giuliano A E, Jones R C, Brennan M, Statman R, Sentinel lymphadenectomy in breast cancer. J Clin Oncol 1997; 15: 2345–2350.

30. Giuliano A E, Kirgan D M, Guenther J M, Morton D L. Lymphatic mapping and sentinel lymphadenectomy for breast cancer. Ann Surg 1994; 220: 391–398.

31. Pijpers R, Meijer S, Hoekstra O S et al. Impact of lymphoscintigraphy on sentinel node identification with technetium-99m-colloidal albumin in breast cancer. J Nucl Med 1997; 38: 366–368.

32. Krag D, Weaver D, Ashikaga T et al. The sentinel node in breast cancer, a multicenter validation study. N Engl J Med 1998; 339: 941–946.

Philip D. Coleridge Smith

Modern approaches to venous disease

Venous diseases of the lower limb veins remain common, affecting about 20% of the adult population of Western countries. In general, these cause no major life threatening illness, and yet the morbidity of venous ulceration places a substantial burden on the community healthcare system and results in the expenditure of large sums on the daily management of this problem. Research continues into better ways to manage venous diseases but, although no great advance has been made in recent years, implementation of currently available technology will result in a better outcome for patients with clinical problems attributable to venous diseases.

VARICOSE VEINS

Varicose veins are managed by a wide range of surgeons who employ numerous different techniques. The major advances which have been made in recent years are in the investigation of venous problems. Clinical examination of patients with venous disease remains useful as an indication of the nature of the clinical problem (distribution of veins, type of veins, presence of skin changes and ulceration). Tourniquet tests add some information about the location of venous valvular incompetence but are notoriously unreliable, even in experienced hands. The information about the function of the veins of the leg gained by these tests is small and insufficient for the management of all but the most simple problems. The state of competence of the superficial veins can be assessed with greater confidence using continuous wave (CW) 'hand-held' Doppler ultrasound. This should be the minimum investigation before undertaking any operation for diseases of the lower limb veins. This allows the competence of the long and short saphenous veins to be assessed with some confidence, although it does not provide accurate anatomical data about the

Mr Philip D. Coleridge Smith DM FRCS, Reader in Surgery, Royal Free and University College Medical School, The Middlesex Hospital, Mortimer Street, London W1N 8AA, UK

location of venous abnormalities. Where previous surgery has been performed, if skin changes or ulceration are present or where the diagnosis is not clear from clinical and CW Doppler examination, an imaging technique should be used. Where a skilled technologist is available with experience in venous imaging, colour duplex ultrasonography is the investigation of choice.[1] All lower limb vessels can be readily assessed using this method providing both anatomical as well as functional information. Alternatively, venography may be employed. However, this is an invasive investigation and, although excellent anatomical detail is provided, functional information is much less satisfactory.

Key point 1

- Assessment by Doppler ultrasound is essential to plan correct treatment.

The treatment recommended depends on the severity of the clinical problem and the expectations of the patient as well as what is possible, judged following objective evaluation of the lower limb veins by CW Doppler or duplex ultrasonography. Some patients simply seek reassurance that their veins will not be the source of fatal pulmonary embolism. Elderly patients may be content to wear medical compression stockings to control symptoms of aching or ankle swelling. Most younger patients prefer to undergo a definitive intervention to remove their veins and this will frequently necessitate surgical treatment.

SURGICAL TREATMENTS

For patients who have large (> 3 mm diameter) varices with or without truncal incompetence of the saphenous veins, surgery should be considered. Where there is a history of previous deep vein thrombosis (DVT) or any clinical feature suggestive of deep vein obstruction or incompetence, the state of the deep veins should be assessed using duplex ultrasonography. In patients in whom the deep veins have been destroyed by a previous DVT, the superficial varices may be the only route of collateral venous drainage. Removing these veins will lead to no symptomatic improvement and may make matters considerably worse. Where deep veins have been damaged by a previous DVT and recanalisation has occurred (demonstrated by duplex ultrasonography), there is no specific contra-indication to varicose vein surgery. However, such patients are at high risk of developing further DVT following varicose vein surgery and will probably derive little symptomatic benefit from surgical removal of varices. In some patients, deep vein incompetence occurs without evidence of previous venous thrombosis but in association with large superficial varices. It has been found that deep vein reflux occurring in these circumstances often resolves when the varicose veins are removed.[2] Patients with primary (non-thrombotic) deep vein incompetence combined with superficial venous incompetence are in the only group in which varicose vein surgery is appropriate.

Key point 2

- Patients with superficial incompetence and varices > 3 mm require surgical treatment. Patients with deep incompetence should only undergo operation if there is no evidence of previous deep vein thrombosis.

The three main principles which should be applied whenever operating to remove varicose veins are first to ligate any incompetent junction or incompetent communication with the deep veins (sapheno-femoral junction [SFJ], sapheno-popliteal junction [SPJ], perforating veins). Next, the associated saphenous trunk is removed (long or short saphenous vein). Finally, all visible varicosities are removed. Most frequently there is only one major source of venous incompetence in a patient with primary varices. However, perhaps 10% of patients have two or more sources of venous reflux. Most commonly, both the sapheno-femoral and sapheno-popliteal junctions are incompetent where there are multiple sources of venous reflux. Failure to ligate all sources of venous reflux during a varicose vein operation will usually result in rapid reappearance of varices. This emphasises the need for reliable pre-operative diagnosis using Doppler ultrasound or duplex ultrasonography. In anatomical locations at which there is significant variation in anatomical position of veins, such as the popliteal fossa, skin marking of the actual location of the SSV and SPJ using an ultrasound imaging machine helps greatly in the identification of these veins at operation (Fig. 1). Thigh and calf perforating veins can also be located using this technique. Care is required in the dissection of the SFJ and SPJ. All tributaries of these junctions should be ligated flush with the vein, leaving none as the source of possible recurrence.

Key point 3

- All sites of deep/superficial incompetence must be identified and ligated.

There has been debate over the years as to the need for stripping the long or short saphenous vein. The increased bruising and risk of cutaneous nerve injury are reasons for not stripping these veins. However, if the SFJ is ligated without stripping the long saphenous vein, the LSV remains patent and incompetent, filling from its tributaries.[3] This results in a higher rate of recurrence than for LSV stripping operations.[4,5] The risk of saphenous nerve injury can be reduced by limiting the stripping procedure to the thigh and upper calf (often called 'short-stripping' by European surgeons). In addition,

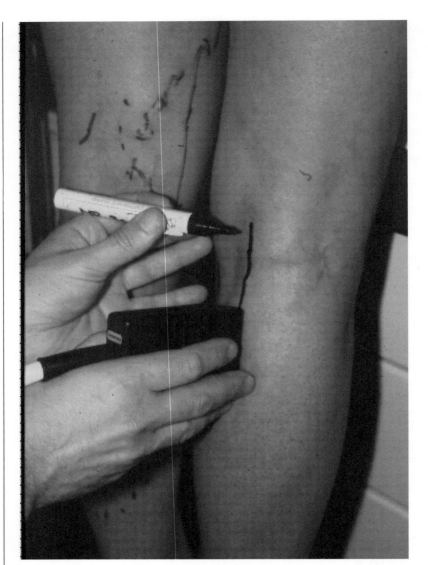

Fig. 1 Ultrasound imaging used to mark the exact position of the short saphenous vein and sapheno-popliteal junction before operation.

use of an inverting stripping method which avoids the use of an olive passed along the track of the vein minimises the risk of nerve injury, bruising and discomfort to the patient.[6,7] Traditionally a flexible stripper wire is passed along the saphenous trunk to remove the vein. This is best passed from the dissected sapheno-femoral or sapheno-popliteal junction distally and recovered in the upper calf, following which the saphenous vein is removed in the same direction. A flexible stripper is not always the best instrument to use for this purpose. It is not easily steered and may pass into a superficial tributary of the saphenous vein, failing to remove the main trunk. It may not be possible to pass it beyond a varicosity in the thigh. Difficulty may be experienced recovering the stripper in the calf, since it will lie deeply in the

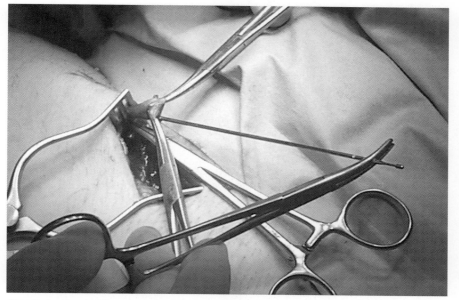

Fig. 2 An Oesch 'Pin-stripper' used to remove the saphenous trunks.

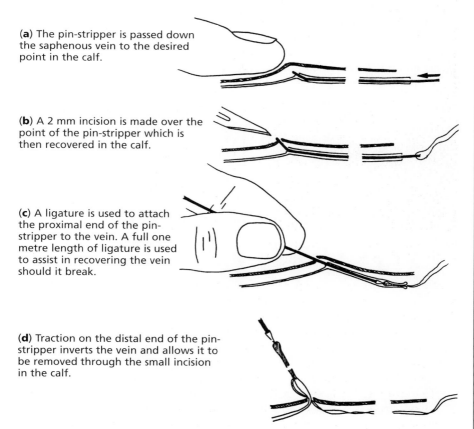

(**a**) The pin-stripper is passed down the saphenous vein to the desired point in the calf.

(**b**) A 2 mm incision is made over the point of the pin-stripper which is then recovered in the calf.

(**c**) A ligature is used to attach the proximal end of the pin-stripper to the vein. A full one metre length of ligature is used to assist in recovering the vein should it break.

(**d**) Traction on the distal end of the pin-stripper inverts the vein and allows it to be removed through the small incision in the calf.

Fig. 3 Inverting stripping techniques used to remove the saphenous vein.

main saphenous trunk. A recently introduced alternative to flexible wire strippers is the Oesch 'pin-stripper'.[8] This is a stiff metal rod 450 mm long with an angulated end which is passed along the vein (Fig. 2). It can be rotated to facilitate steering into the desired vein and is easily recovered through a 3 mm incision in the calf. It is specifically designed to be used for inverting stripping of the saphenous veins (Fig. 3), a method originally described by Keller in 1905.[9]

Key point 4

- Techniques exist for stripping venous trunks with minimal trauma and small incisions. All affected venous trunks should be stripped.

The final part of the operative procedure is to remove all visible varicosities. Traditionally, incisions were made and forceps introduced to remove the varicosities and the incision was sutured. This results in large, unsightly scars in the leg which often have a poor cosmetic appearance. 'Hook phlebectomy' is now widely practised and allows varices to be removed through very small incisions resulting in an excellent cosmetic outcome. Several different designs of hook are available and the most appropriate will depend on personal preference. The author prefers Oesch hooks which can be introduced through incisions of 1–2 mm in length (Fig. 4). These recover all small to large size

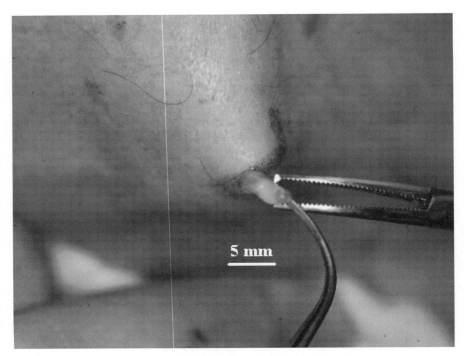

5 mm

Fig. 4 Oesch phlebectomy hook used to retrieve superficial varices.

varices with great success. Occasionally, very large varices are difficult to capture using a hook and have to be seized with a forceps. 'Micro-Halsteads' fine toothed artery forceps are as small as mosquito clips, but have the added advantage of possessing teeth. The aim is to grasp the vein with either a hook or micro-Halsteads forceps and bring it to the surface. A large artery forceps can then be applied and, with gentle traction, several centimetres of vein can be removed. Incisions of 1–2 mm in length must be made along the track of all varices to be removed. The intervals between incisions depend on the length of the varicose vein retrieved from each incision. Incisions of small dimensions require no suturing and may be covered with 'Steristrips' or simple adhesive wound dressings.

Postoperative management includes the use of compression stockings or bandages. There is reliable evidence to show that crepe and elastocrepe bandages have poor elastic properties.[10] Modern bandages and stockings have far superior compressive ability and many surgeons now use these as the method of compressing the limb. The use of class 2 medical compression stockings worn for 1–3 weeks postoperatively is widespread practice in the UK at present.

Key point 5

- All visible varices should be excised through incisions 1–2 mm in length.

THE MANAGEMENT OF SMALL VARICES AND TELANGIECTASES

Many patients present in surgical clinics with varices of < 3 mm diameter, including telangiectases (thread veins, spider veins) of the lower limbs. Varices of small diameter usually lie just beneath the skin and are referred to as reticular veins. These are associated with incompetence of the long or short saphenous vein in about 30% of cases, so it is worthwhile investigating whether the saphenous trunks are competent using CW Doppler or duplex ultrasonography. It is usually advisable to remove the incompetent long or short saphenous vein where it communicates with and fills these small varices. Reticular veins of larger diameter (2–3 mm) can be removed surgically using small vein hooks. However, many patients have the combination of reticular veins and telangiectases. The cosmetic improvement achieved by surgical treatment in such patients is negligible. In fact, in patients with telangiectases, surgical intervention often results in the development of still more telangiectases, since any damage to the skin causes the abnormal angiogenesis which results in the formation of telangiectases. By far the most effective treatment for patients with telangiectases and reticular veins in the absence of superficial venous incompetence is microsclerotherapy. In this technique, the telangiectases and reticular veins are injected directly using a fine needle (usually 30 g) and a suitable sclerosant of low concentration. The method and sclerosant differ greatly from those used to treat truncal varices and are best

Key point 6

- Microsclerotherapy can improve the appearance of legs affected by telangiectasia and reticular veins.

learned from a skilled practitioner of this technique. A note of warning: 3% STD, which is widely used to inject large varices, results in severe damage to the skin when injected into thread veins. Treatment for telangiectases carried out correctly will remove 80–90% of visible veins. Patients often think that laser treatment is appropriate for the management of leg veins. This is partially correct in that a suitable laser will remove telangiectases. Reticular veins are beyond the scope of lasers and still have to be injected. In addition, laser treatment usually progresses more slowly, and perhaps more painfully than microsclerotherapy in the lower limbs. For telangiectases of the face and upper trunk laser treatment is superior to injection treatments. Treatment of small veins has been extensively discussed in a recent monograph.[11]

RECURRENT VARICOSE VEINS

A detailed knowledge of the anatomy of recurrent varices is required before they can be reliably treated. This is best done using duplex ultrasonography, although some surgeons prefer the images of recurrent varices obtained by venography.[12] This method is becoming much less widely used than previously. The most frequent cause of recurrent varices following surgery to the SFJ is further varices arising from the SFJ.[13] This is caused by residual tributaries or poor surgical technique in the original operation. In some patients, it appears that neovascularisation accounts for the recurrent varices.[14] Further surgery in this region requires a careful approach. A lateral approach allows the femoral artery to be identified with confidence. Usually this area has not been dissected previously. Subsequently, the region of dissection passes medially to the femoral vein, allowing visualisation of the SFJ. In patients who have previously been treated by sapheno-femoral ligation without stripping of the long saphenous vein, this should be removed at the operation. It may be possible to identify the residual vein in the groin. Alternatively, it can usually be easily found as it passes the knee. A stripper passed along the vein allows it to be removed by an inverting technique or a conventional method.

The sapheno-popliteal junction is more difficult to dissect a second time since the several motor and sensory nerves in this region are easily damaged leading to far worse problems than the original veins. Considerable caution

Key point 7

- Surgery for recurrent varicose veins may be difficult and requires full anatomical information.

Table 1 Conditions other than venous disease that may cause ulceration of the lower limb

Peripheral arterial disease
Diabetes mellitus
Peripheral neuropathy
Rheumatoid disease
Leg trauma
Malignant skin ulcers
Basal cell carcinomas
Squamous cell carcinomas
Malignant melanomas
Systemic inflammatory disorders resulting in vasculitis
Systemic lupus erythematosus
Systemic sclerosis

should be used in re-exploring the popliteal fossa, preferably placing any new incision away from sites of previous surgery. The anatomy of the recurrent veins should be investigated using duplex ultrasonography to assess the difficulty of the task.

VENOUS ULCERATION

This condition remains a common problem in medical practice. The prevalence of skin changes of the limb which precedes leg ulceration is about 1–2% of the adult population of Western countries. At any one time, about 0.25% of the population suffer from leg ulceration.[15,16] The cost of this is considerable and has been estimated at £400–600 million per annum in the UK. A large element of this problem is the cost of managing ulcers in the community. Community nursing staff spend as much as half their time attending to patients with leg ulceration. Far lesser amounts are expended on hospital treatment these days. Leg ulceration is associated with venous disease in about 60–70% of cases, but a wide range of conditions may also cause leg ulcers (Table 1).

The management of leg ulcers has been greatly assisted by the availability of duplex ultrasonography. It has been found, in a number of studies, that a large proportion of patients with a venous cause for their leg ulcer have superficial venous incompetence alone, that is they have varicose ulcers.[17] It is well known that many leg ulcers heal following treatment of varicose veins. Using duplex ultrasonography, this group of patients can be reliably identified and offered surgical treatment. These ulcers usually heal rapidly and remain healed following surgical treatment with a low annual recurrence rate.

Those patients with deep vein incompetence usually fare less well. Deep vein incompetence is often caused by previous venous thrombosis. In some patients, deep vein incompetence is found without evidence of previous thrombosis. These conditions can be recognised, to some extent during duplex ultrasonography. For these patients, there is no advantage in removing superficial varices, even if any are present. The mainstay of treatment here should be compression treatments.

COMPRESSION TREATMENT

In the UK, compression stockings are available in three grades of compression: class 1, 2 and 3 compression stockings. For patients with venous ulceration, class 2 or 3 compression is the most appropriate. Stockings can be used successfully over a dressing, provided that it is well taped to the skin. Patients who have never received compression treatment often heal swiftly in response to moderate levels of compression. The use of compression stockings necessitates fairly strong hands and arms. Many elderly patients are too frail to use stockings, and bandages must be employed instead. The 4-layer technique of bandaging is now widely taught to nurses involved in the management of leg ulcers. The first two layers (wool and crepe) pad the limb sufficiently to allow 45 mmHg compression to be applied. The final two layers apply enough compression to heal 70% of ulcers in 12 weeks.[18] It is important when applying compression to ensure that significant arterial disease is not present, otherwise severe ischaemic complications of treatment could ensue. Although ulcer healing can readily be achieved in most patients if high enough levels of compression can be tolerated, recurrence of ulceration is common after healing achieved in this way. As many as 25% of patients suffer recurrence every year following healing achieved by compression bandaging.[19] The prevention of recurrent ulceration remains a significant problem that has yet to be fully addressed. Those patients who wear strong compression stockings following healing fare better than those who do not.

Key point 8

- Most patients with venous ulcers will respond to compression treatment; continued compression helps reduce recurrence.

Whilst the factors which lead to venous ulcer healing are widely under-stood, they are not always incorporated into treatment for patients. It has been shown that systematically organised clinics in hospitals or in the community in which all medical and nursing personnel involved in the management of patients use the best available techniques of compression can achieve high rates of healing.[20]

SURGICAL TREATMENT

A number of surgical procedures have been described for patients with severe symptoms attributable to their vein problems. The deep veins can be repaired if the valves are incompetent. Where no previous venous thrombosis has occurred and symptoms are attributable to primary venous incompetence, surgery can be carried out to the valve cusps to restore normal function. If the valves have been destroyed by previous venous thrombosis, then a valve can be taken with the axillary vein and this can be transposed to the incompetent segment in the lower limb. In practice, these operations would only be considered in relatively young patients with severe symptoms. The scale of surgery is far greater than would be appropriate in an elderly, frail patient.

Perforating veins were once thought to be the entire problem in patients with severe venous disease. Operations to ligate them were performed in the expectation of achieving long-term healing of leg ulcers. This surgery was often carried out contemporaneously with standard varicose vein surgery. In many patients this led to long-term ulcer healing. In others, very poor healing or even severe postoperative complications would ensue with infection of the operation site and extension of the ulcer. It has been shown that, where deep vein damage is present, conventional perforating vein surgery does not prevent ulcer recurrence or improve venous physiological function in the lower limb.[21,22] This subject has been revisited with the advent of endoscopic techniques. It is now possible to ligate medial calf perforating veins without the need to make incisions in the region of the skin damaged by lipodermato-sclerosis.[23,24] It has been shown that, in combination with superficial venous surgery, sub-fascial endoscopic perforator surgery (SEPS) achieves healing of venous ulcers. It is not clear from any study so far published whether there is any advantage to patients with deep vein incompetence of having this procedure performed. Some serious complications of the procedure have been described; saphenous nerve injury is common and tibial nerve damage has been described in a number of patients.[25] In German speaking countries, it is common practice to perform a closed para-tibial fasciotomy of the superficial posterior compartment of the leg at the same time as endoscopic perforating vein surgery.[26] There is no reliable study to support this technique. Despite this, it is widely practised and several large clinical series have been published.

Key point 9

- Operations to ligate incompetent perforations will help only the small number of patients with a normal deep system. Other patients should have compression therapy.

In summary, superficial venous surgery is appropriate in up to half of the patients who present with a venous ulcer since they have superficial venous incompetence alone. In a few patients, isolated perforating vein incompetence is present (with normal deep veins). These can be ligated with advantage. In patients with deep vein incompetence as a consequence of a previous DVT it is unlikely that superficial or perforating vein surgery will offer any advantage. In a small proportion of young patients with severe symptoms due to their venous disease, deep vein reconstruction can be considered. These are technically difficult procedures performed in only a few centres with an uncertain long-term outlook, although some authors have reported satisfactory results.[27,28]

THE CAUSES OF VENOUS ULCERATION

It has been recognised that patients who develop venous ulceration have impairment of the calf venous pump and this results in persistently raised

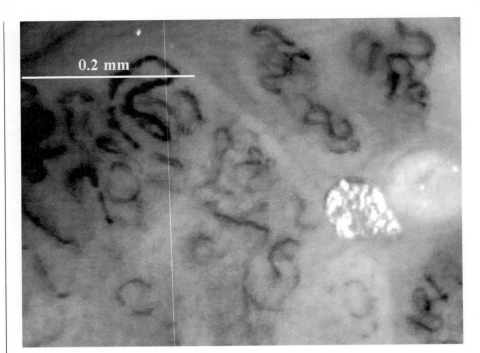

Fig. 5 Dilated and convoluted skin capillaries seen through a capillary microscope in lipodermatosclerotic skin in a patient with venous disease. The analogy with a glomerulus is easily seen.

venous pressure in the superficial veins which is not decreased during walking. The venous pressure on standing still is not abnormal in patients with leg ulcers. In practice, a wide range of ambulatory venous pressures is observed and, even if more recent methods of measurement are used, a large scatter of data is obtained. This may partially reflect inadequacies of the measurement systems but is also attributable to differences in individual patient susceptibility to venous ulceration.

The mechanisms which result in venous ulceration have yet to be fully elucidated. The research which has been conducted in this area has been reviewed in detail in two recent monographs.[29,30] It has been known for some time that the focus of skin damage which eventually results in leg ulceration lies in the papillary capillaries. These vessels become convoluted and resemble glomeruli (Fig. 5). They are surrounded by a complex inflammatory reaction and this seems to cause extensive fibrosis in the skin and subcutaneous fat. Leukocytes become sequestered in the lower limbs during periods of venous hypertension and it is proposed that these cells adhere to the capillary or post-capillary venule endothelium and initiate the injury sequence. Leukocyte-endothelial cell interactions are strongly determined by flow rates in the capillaries and venules. It has been shown that compression stockings prevent sequestration of leukocytes in the lower limb during venous hypertension. Compression applied to the skin appears to accelerate flow in the microcirculation deterring leukocytes from adhering to endothelial cells. This is a possible mechanism by which compression protects the microcirculation of the skin from damage and achieves leg ulcer healing in patients with venous disease.

DRUG TREATMENT

In the UK, very few drugs are prescribed in the management of venous diseases. No drug currently available will cure varicose veins. However, varicose veins give rise to a wide range of symptoms ranging from aching and ankle oedema to restless legs and cramps. In many European countries, these symptoms are treated using 'venotonic' drugs. These are largely derived from plant extracts and fall into a number of chemical groups including aescin, rutin, hydroxyrutosides, flavonoids. In the UK, only hydroxyrutosides are available as Paroven (Zyma, Switzerland). Venotonic drugs have been found to relieve the symptoms of venous disease including ankle oedema.

Key point 10

- No drug therapy has been shown to be as good as compression therapy for the healing of venous ulcers.

Venous ulcers still prove to be a difficult problem as far as pharmacotherapy is concerned. A number of drugs has been investigated but none has been found to be especially active in venous ulceration. Pentoxifylline (Trental, Hoechst-Marion-Roussell) has been investigated in detail. In one clinical study improved healing was found,[31] but when higher levels of compression were applied, statistical significance was lost. Hydroxyrutosides do not prevent venous ulcer recurrence. Aspirin was found to improve ulcer healing in a small study. Ifetroban (Bristol-Myers-Squibb, USA), a thromboxane A_2 receptor antagonist (platelet inhibitor) was ineffective in achieving ulcer healing.[32] One of the venotonic drugs, Daflon (hesperidine and diosmin, Servier) has been shown to benefit ulcer healing in a small study.[33] To date, no drug has been found which equals the efficacy of strong compression bandages (70% healing in 12 weeks). Research continues to elucidate the mechanisms which are involved in producing ulcers which might be addressed by drug treatments.

Many topical applications have been used to dress leg ulcers. None has been shown conclusively to speed leg ulcer healing. Hydrocolloid wound dressings achieve the same healing rate as do non-adherent dressings. Tissue growth factors applied topically once promised much in speeding ulcer healing, but properly conducted clinical trials have shown no effect in achieving wound healing.[34]

The perfect drug to treat venous ulceration has yet to be devised. A number of potential pathological mechanisms could be addressed. At present, investigation of these will be largely based on empirical principles. An advantage of finding a drug active in healing venous ulceration will be that it may address the underlying cause of ulceration and allow treatment to be given which will prevent recurrence.

SUMMARY

Venous diseases are common and are widely encountered in surgical practice. Modern methods of treating varicose veins ensure that all sources of varices can be detected and veins can be removed through inconspicuous incisions. Small varices can be treated effectively by sclerotherapy. Venous ulceration often arises in patients with superficial venous incompetence alone. All patients presenting with leg ulceration or severe skin changes deserve to be investigated by duplex ultrasonography if they would be fit enough for superficial venous surgery. Patients with superficial venous incompetence alone or isolated perforating incompetence should be offered operation. Young patients with severe symptoms could be referred to a specialist unit with view to deep vein reconstruction, if this is feasible. Compression treatment remains effective in the management of venous ulceration and should be the primary treatment in all other patients with venous leg ulceration. No drug is as effective as good compression in achieving healing. No topical treatment,

Key points for clinical practice

- .Assessment by Doppler ultrasound is essential to plan correct treatment.
- Patients with superficial incompetence and varices > 3 mm require surgical treatment. Patients with deep incompetence should only undergo operation if there is no evidence of previous deep vein thrombosis.
- All sites of deep/superficial incompetence must be identified and ligated.
- Techniques exist for stripping venous trunks with minimal trauma and small incisions. All affected venous trunks should be stripped.
- All visible varices should be excised through incisions 1–2 mm in length.
- Microsclerotherapy can improve the appearance of legs affected by telangiectasia and reticular veins.
- Surgery for recurrent varicose veins may be difficult and requires full anatomical information.
- Most patients with venous ulcers will respond to compression treatment; continued compression helps reduce recurrence.
- Operations to ligate incompetent perforations will help only the small number of patients with a normal deep system. Other patients should have compression therapy.
- No drug therapy has been shown to be as good as compression therapy for the healing of venous ulcers.

whether simple or active, speeds ulcer healing. Recurrence following healing remains a problem. All patients who have been treated with compression to achieve healing should be encouraged to wear medical compression stockings to prevent recurrence.

References

1. Mercer K G, Scott D J, Berridge D C. Preoperative duplex imaging is required before all operations for primary varicose veins. Br J Surg 1998; 85: 1495–1497.
2. Walsh J C, Bergan J J, Beeman S, Comer T P. Femoral venous reflux abolished by greater saphenous vein stripping. Ann Vasc Surg 1994; 8: 566–570.
3. McMullin G M, Coleridge Smith P D, Scurr J H. Objective assessment of high ligation without stripping of the long saphenous vein. Br J Surg 1991; 78: 1139–1142.
4. Sarin S, Scurr J H, Coleridge Smith P D. Stripping of the long saphenous vein in the treatment of primary varicose veins. Br-J-Surg 1994; 81: 1455–1458.
5. Jones M, Braithwaite B D, Selwyn D, Cooke S, Earnshaw J J. Neovascularisation is the principal cause of varicose vein recurrence: results of a randomised trial of stripping the long saphenous vein. Eur J Vasc Endovasc Surg 1996; 12: 442–445.
6. Van der Stricht J. Saphencetomie sur fil. Presse Med Paris 1963; 71: 1081–1082.
7. Ouvry P A. Stripping par invagination sur mèche calibrée. Phlébologie 1989; 42: 599–604.
8. Oesch A. 'Pin-stripping': a novel method of atraumatic stripping. Phlebology 1993; 8: 171–173.
9. Keller W L. A new method of extirpating the internal saphenous and similar veins in varicose conditions; a preliminary report. NY Med J 1905; 82: 385.
10 Coleridge Smith P D, Scurr J H. Optimum methods of limb compression following varicose vein surgery. Phlebology 1987; 2: 165–172.
11. Goldman M, Weiss R, Bergan J J. (eds) Varicose Veins and Telangiectasias: Diagnosis and Treatment, 2nd edn. St Louis, MO: Quality Medical Publishing, 1998.
12 Stonebridge P A, Chalmers N, Beggs I, Bradbury A W, Ruckley C V. Recurrent varicose veins: a varicographic analysis leading to a new practical classification. Br J Surg 1995; 82: 60–62.
13. Redwood N F, Lambert D. Patterns of reflux in recurrent varicose veins assessed by duplex scanning. Br J Surg 1994; 81: 1450–1451.
14. Nyamekye I, Shephard N A, Davies B, Heather B P, Earnshaw J J. Clinicopathological evidence that neovascularisation is a cause of recurrent varicose veins. Eur J Vasc Endovasc Surg 1998; 15: 412–415.
15. Nelzen O, Bergqvist D, Lindhagen A. Venous and non venous leg ulcers: clinical history and appearance in a population study. Br J Surg 1994; 81: 182–187.
16. Baker S R, Stacey M C, Jopp McKay A G, Hoskin S E, Thompson P J. Epidemiology of chronic venous ulcers. Br J Surg 1991; 78: 864–867.
17. Scriven J M, Hartshorne T, Thrush A J, Bell P R, Naylor A R, London N J. Role of saphenous vein surgery in the treatment of venous ulceration. Br J Surg 1998; 85: 781–784.
18. Moffatt C J, Franks P J, Oldroyd M et al. Community clinics for leg ulcers and impact on healing. BMJ 1992; 305: 1389–1392.
19. Franks P J, Oldroyd M I, Dickson D, Sharp E J, Moffatt C J. Risk factors for leg ulcer recurrence: a randomized trial of two types of compression stocking. Age Ageing 1995; 24: 490–494.
20. Ghauri A S, Nyamekye I, Grabs A J, Farndon J R, Whyman M R, Poskitt K R Influence of a specialised leg ulcer service and venous surgery on the outcome of venous leg ulcers. Eur J Vasc Endovasc Surg 1998; 16: 238–244.
21. Burnand K G, Lea Thomas M, O'Donnell T, Browse N L. Relation between postphlebitic changes in deep veins and results of surgical treatment of venous ulcers. Lancet 1976; i: 936–938.
22. Stacey M C, Burnand K G, Layer G T, Pattison M. Calf pump function in patients with healed venous ulcers is not improved by surgery to the communicating veins or by elastic stockings. Br J Surg 1988; 75: 436–439.

23. Gloviczki P, Bergan J J, Menawat S S et al. Safety, feasibility, and early efficacy of subfascial endoscopic perforator surgery: a preliminary report from the North American registry. J Vasc Surg 1997; 25: 94–105.

24. Pierik E G, van Urk H, Wittens C H. Efficacy of subfascial endoscopy in eradicating perforating veins of the lower leg and its relation with venous ulcer healing. J Vasc Surg 1997; 26: 255–259.

25. Whiteley M S, Smith J J, Galland R B. Tibial nerve damage during subfascial endoscopic perforator vein surgery. Br J Surg 1997; 84: 512.

26. Vanderpuye R. Die paratibiale Fasziotomie. Wien Med Wochenschr 1994; 144: 262–263.

27. Raju S, Fredericks R K, Neglen P N, Bass J D Durability of venous valve reconstruction techniques for 'primary' and postthrombotic reflux. J Vasc Surg 1996; 23: 357–366.

28. Masuda E M; Kistner R L. Long-term results of venous valve reconstruction: a four- to twenty-one-year follow-up. J Vasc Surg 1994; 19: 391–403.

29 Coleridge Smith P D. (ed) The Microcirculation in Venous Disease. Austin, TX: Landes, 1998.

30 Messmer K. (ed) Progress in Applied Microcirculation, Vol. 23. Microcirculation in chronic venous insufficiency. Munich: Karger, 1999.

31. Colgan M-P, Dormandy J A, Jones P W, Schraibman I G, Shanik D G. Oxpentifyline treatment of venous ulcers of the leg. BMJ 1990; 300: 972–975.

32. Lyon R T, Veith F J, Bolton L, Machado F. Clinical benchmark for healing of chronic venous ulcers. Venous Ulcer Study Collaborators (IFETROBAN study). Am J Surg 1998; 176: 172–175.

33. Guilhou J J, Dereure O, Marzin L et al. Efficacy of Daflon 500 mg in venous leg ulcer healing: a double-blind, randomised, controlled versus placebo trial in 107 patients. Angiology 1997; 48; 77–85.

34. Falanga V, Eaglstein W H, Bucalo B, Katz M H, Harris B, Carson P. Topical use of human recombinant epidermal growth factor (hEGF) in venous ulcers. J Dermatol Surg Oncol 1992; 18: 604–606.

A. M. H. Amin I. Taylor

What's new in general surgery – a review of the journals

This chapter attempts to emphasise and highlight the key publications in the field of general surgery. It reviews the reported advances in the management of surgical problems. The chapter is divided into upper gastrointestinal surgery, lower gastrointestinal surgery, hepatopancreatobiliary surgery, and breast surgery, and endocrine surgery.

UPPER GASTROINTESTINAL DISEASES

GASTRO-OESOPHAGEAL REFLUX

One-third to one-half of patients presenting with chest pain have no evidence of coronary artery disease and are characterised as having non-cardiac chest pain. In a large subset of these patients, the oesophagus might be the source of the symptoms. Demedts et al[1] have summarised recent progress in the understanding of chest pain of oesophageal origin. Symptomatic gastroesophageal reflux is the most common cause and the use of impedance planimetry has provided a better insight into the mechanisms underlying hypersensitivity to oesophageal balloon distension. The high prevalence and likely role of panic disorder in patients with chest pain of non-cardiac origin has been confirmed. Further investigations towards factors underlying atypical chest pain should include not only a gastrointestinal but also a psychological work-up.

It is unclear why some patients with columnar-lined oesophagus present with intestinal metaplasia and others do not. The pathophysiological and

Mr A.M.H. Amin FRCS FRCS (Glasg), Senior Registrar and Lecturer, Department of Surgery, Royal Free University College Medical School London, Charles Bell House, 67–73 Riding House Street, London W1P 7LD, UK

Prof. I. Taylor MD ChM FRCS, Professor of Surgery and Head of Department of Surgery, Royal Free University College Medical School London, Charles Bell House, 67–73 Riding House Street, London W1P 7LD, UK

clinical implications of the length of the metaplastic segment are also controversial. Whether the length of the metaplasia and the presence of intestinal epithelium are related to the clinical, manometric and pH data in patients with columnar-lined oesophagus has been studied.[2] No significant difference was found in any of the variables analysed except for associated inflammatory lesions above the columnar epithelium, which were more frequent in patients with a shorter metaplastic segment. Neither the length of the metaplastic segment nor the presence of intestinal metaplasia were related to more advanced gastro-oesophageal reflux disease or to poorer oesophageal clearing function or to higher acid reflux rates.

GASTRO-OESOPHAGEAL REFLUX SURGERY

In a comparison between laparoscopic and open surgery in the treatment of gastro-oesophageal reflux disease, 80 patients with gastro-oesophageal reflux disease underwent laparoscopic surgical treatment.[3] All cases were studied pre-operatively with endoscopy, manometry and pH monitoring. Both laparoscopic and open techniques were found to offer good results. However, open surgical procedures have a higher morbidity (18% versus 6.7%); therefore, the laparoscopic approach should be considered a safer technique. Anvari et al[4] have also reported that laparoscopic Nissen fundoplication is an effective antireflux procedure at 2 years follow-up with satisfactory long-term results.

OESOPHAGEAL CANCER

Definitive staging of oesophageal cancer facilitates allocation of patients to appropriate treatment regimens. Thoracoscopy is an excellent means for staging the chest and mediastinum. Lymph node staging for oesophageal cancer, by both thoracoscopic and laparoscopic approaches, have been used since 1992 and are more accurate than existing staging methods.[5] The value of laparoscopy and laparoscopic ultrasonography in the staging of oesophageal and cardial carcinoma was also reported by Romijin et al.[6] However, neither was found to be effective for oesophageal carcinoma although, in carcinoma of the cardia, laparoscopy was more effective, especially when combined with laparoscopic ultrasonography. Bronchoscopy has also been used as a staging tool to assess invasion of oesophageal cancer into the tracheobronchial tree.[7]

Long-term survival rates following radical oesophagectomy are poor. Surgery remains the mainstay of radical treatment. Sykes et al[8] have shown a survival improvement after radiotherapy similar for both squamous cell and adenocarcinoma.

Recurrence of thoracic oesophageal carcinoma in the cervical and superior mediastinal lymph nodes occurs frequently and contributes to a poor prognosis. In a prospective randomised trial of extended and conventional lymphadenectomy, Nishihira et al demonstrated possible prevention of recurrence and prolongation of survival.[9]

There is growing evidence that blood transfusion is associated with immuno-suppression. The effect of peri-operative allogeneic blood transfusion on survival was studied retrospectively in 524 patients who were discharged from the hospital after oesophago-gastrectomy. Although peri-operative allogeneic blood transfusion does not affect long-term survival after oesophago-gastrectomy for carcinoma, it does have a significant association with short-term survival in a group whose overall survival is often limited after resection. Attention, therefore, should be directed toward minimising operative blood loss and the subsequent blood transfusion requirement.[10]

UPPER GASTROINTESTINAL BLEEDING

Chow et al[11] looked at the risk factors for rebleeding and death from peptic ulcer in the elderly. For patients aged 80 years or older, the significant factors were ulcer size greater than 2 cm and admission with serum bilirubin above 20 mmol/l. Endoscopic treatment for the elderly was effective if carried out early.

In a randomised controlled trial, endoscopic injection of bleeding oeso-phageal varices with either sclerotherapy or fibrin glue were compared.[12] Rebleeding, especially during the first 28 days, was less common in the fibrin group, and all patients treated with fibrin glue survived for more than 28 days. In contrast, 5 patients treated with polidocanol died within this period. The incidence of sclerotherapy-induced ulcers was significantly lower in the fibrin group than in the polidocanol group, and major complications such as perforation or ulcer bleeding were observed only in the polidocanol group. Therefore, fibrin glue is an efficient and safe agent for endoscopic sclerotherapy of bleeding oesophageal varices.

Endoscopic detachable mini-loop ligation is a simple and safe procedure for treatment of oesophageal varices.[13] Application of mini-loops does not induce uncontrolled bleeding; however, it may induce superficial ulceration at ligation sites.

GASTRIC CANCER

Sanchez et al,[14] in a multivariate analysis, reported that gastric wall invasion, lymph node invasion, tumour size and dysphagia at presentation were the only independent prognostic variables following surgical resection. From these data, it could be possible to derive a prognostic index by which patients could be classified at low, intermediate or high risk.

The effect of pre-operative chemotherapy in downgrading locally advanced unresectable gastric cancer has been evaluated.[15] Patients received weekly cisplatin, 5-fluorouracil, epidoxorubicin, 6S-stereoisomer of leucovorin and glutathione in addition to filgrastim by subcutaneous injection. This intensive regimen enabled resection in half of previously inoperable tumours with a moderate toxicity.

Infection with *Helicobacter pylori* has been designated a cause of human cancer by the International Agency for Research on Cancer.[16] Populations at high risk of gastric cancer have a high prevalence of *H. pylori* infection. Individuals with antibodies to *H. pylori* were more likely to develop gastric cancer, and the relative risk after an interval of 15 or more years was 8.7 compared with seronegative subjects.

Surgical technique

A number of papers have reported the results of surgical treatments for different stages of gastric cancer. Limited resection for early gastric cancer of the upper stomach (EGCUS) without lymph node metastasis was discussed and evaluated by Furukawa et al.[17] Since 1988, a total of 34 patients with EGCUS have undergone a limited operation (fundectomy) which includes a limited proximal gastrectomy, a limited lymph node dissection, and a procedure preserving the vagal nerve. The surgical risk, postoperative complications, and survival rates of the fundectomy patients were compared with those undergoing total gastrectomy. A limited fundectomy for EGCUS has decreased the surgical risk and postoperative complications without decreasing the survival rate.

The influence of extended (D2) lymph node dissection on gastric cancer survival was also assessed by Roukos et al.[18] Survival data of patients with involved nodes (N2 disease) was evaluated. The 5-year survival rate for the N2 patients was 17%, overall hospital mortality and morbidity were 1.3% and 33.4%, respectively. It was, therefore, felt that D2 resection can be performed safely and is of therapeutic value in patients with advanced lymph node metastases. The outcome of D2 resections for gastric cancer in Western patients was also evaluated by Degiuli et al.[19] The more extensive Japanese procedure with pancreas preservation was found to be a safe radical treatment for gastric cancer for selected Western patients treated in experienced centres. The overall morbidity rate was 20.9%. Surgical complications were observed in 16.7% of patients. Overall mortality rate was 13.6% and a complication rate of 31.2% followed these procedures. The 5-year survival rate for all patients who underwent combined gastrectomy with adjacent organs was 25%. Therefore, advanced gastric cancer should not be considered unresectable.[20]

After total gastrectomy, sustaining good nutrition is extremely important for quality of life. The use of a modified interposition double jejunal pouch following total gastrectomy was evaluated.[21] This technique results in a complete pouch and uses a double stapling technique with anastomosis between the oesophagus and pouch. There were no anastamotic leaks and pouch blood flow was within normal expected limits. After 2 years, mean body-weight was 98.3% of expected, mean food volume was 94.0% of expected and mean meal frequency was 3.0 per day.

BREAST DISEASE

BREAST CANCER

Two interesting studies have looked at the effects of chronic stress and menstrual cycle on breast cancer progression. Stress can effect the immune system with possible reduction in disease progression and metastatic spread. Andersen et al[22] demonstrated in 116 patients that the physiological effects of stress inhibit cellular immune responses relevant to cancer prognosis. Tumour expression of genes that may contribute to proliferative capacity and metastatic potential can change during the course of the menstrual cycle. Saad et al[23] have suggested that this could provide a molecular explanation for improved survival in patients whose tumours were removed during the luteal phase of the menstrual cycle.

Colditz reviewed the role of hormone replacement therapy in the development of breast cancer.[24] Evidence of a causal relationship between female hormones and breast cancer was explored. The magnitude of the increase in breast cancer risk per year of hormone use is comparable to that associated with delaying menopause by a year. It was also speculated that, hormones may act to promote the late stages of carcinogenesis among postmenopausal women and to facilitate the proliferation of malignant cells.

Hereditary breast cancer has been associated with mutation in the *BRCA1* and *BRCA2* genes and has a natural history different from sporadic breast cancer. Disease free and overall survival were found to be similar for sporadic and hereditary breast cancer with a proven *BRCA1* alteration.[25]

Prevention of breast cancer

It has been suggested tamoxifen may prevent the occurrence of breast cancer. Powles et al[26] have undertaken a trial of tamoxifen in healthy women aged 30–70 years at increased risk of breast cancer because of family history. Individuals were randomised in a double blind fashion to receive tamoxifen 20 mg/day orally or placebo for up to 8 years. They were unable to show any effect of tamoxifen on breast-cancer incidence in healthy women. Similarly, the postulated protective effect of tamoxifen was not apparent in another study.[27] Interestingly enough, women using hormone-replacement therapy appear to benefit from the use of tamoxifen.

Breast screening

Retrospective analysis of all patients with invasive lobular breast cancer, detected by breast cancer screening compared to those detected outside the screening project, have shown that 2, 5, 10 year disease-free survival rate in the screen-detected group was 100%, 100% and 89%, respectively.[28] For the group outside the screening programme this was 88.4%, 74.3% and 72.5%, respectively. No patient in the screen-detected group died from breast cancer during follow-up, whereas the 2, 5, 10 year breast cancer survival rate for the group detected outside the screening programme was 96.5%, 89.1% and 70.6%, respectively. These data suggest that patients in the screen-detected group may have a favourable outcome compared with those who have invasive lobular breast cancer detected outside the screening programme.

Surgical technique

There has been a gradual shift away from radical surgery towards conservation treatment for breast cancer. Pectoralis minor muscle is increasingly preserved in women undergoing axillary clearance. A retrospective study was conducted to determine the axillary node count in 578 patients who underwent axillary clearance, 276 with removal of pectoralis minor and 302 who had the muscle preserved.[29] The mean number of nodes excised in the group who had pectoralis minor excised was 25.5 (range 8–50) compared with 24.5 (range 9–68) in the preservation group. For the majority of patients with operable breast cancer, retention of pectoralis minor muscle was not associated with understaging or undertreatment of the axilla.

The feasibility and benefit of preserving the intercostobrachial nerve (ICBN) to prevent sensory loss was also studied prospectively.[30] Sensory symptoms and deficits were documented, and shoulder movement and arm circumference were measured at discharge and 3 months later in 120 patients randomised to either preservation or division of the ICBN. Preserving the ICBN reduced the incidence of sensory deficit but not sensory symptoms.

Assessment of completion of tumour excision has become an integral part of breast-conserving surgery, but the accuracy of margin analysis has been questioned. The results of resection margin analysis were compared with examination of tumour bed biopsies and of the excised cavity wall.[31] Margin analysis of wide local excision specimens is a poor predictor of completeness of excision without examination of the entire cavity wall. The latter may increase the detection of residual disease compared with examination of bed biopsies alone and is a useful adjuvant to conventional margin evaluation.

Finally, pre-operative prediction of the nipple and areola involvement in breast cancer was addressed by Vyas et al.[32] Areola-tumour distance was measured in 140 patients undergoing mastectomy. The nipple was involved in 22 (16%) patients and in each the tumour was within 2.5 cm of the areola.

Sentinel node biopsy

Sentinel lymph node biopsy is a recently developed, minimally invasive technique for staging the axilla in patients with breast cancer. A wide range of different methods and materials has been employed, but there has been little consensus on the most reliable and reproducible technique. In a comprehensive review, sentinel node biopsy was identified as a valid technique in breast cancer management, which provides valuable axillary staging information.[33] The optimal technique of lymphatic mapping is a combination of vital blue dye and radiolabelled colloid. This technique allows selective axillary dissection in node-positive patients and reduces the need for axillary dissection without compromising survival and regional control[34,35] (*see* Chapter 10).

Adjuvant therapy

Uncontrolled studies suggest that high-dose chemotherapy is beneficial in patients with breast cancer and multiple axillary lymph node metastases. High-dose adjuvant chemotherapy was evaluated in a randomised trial.[36] Although no patients died from the toxic effects of chemotherapy, with a median follow-up of 49 months, there was no significant difference in survival between patients on conventional therapy and those on high-dose therapy. Furthermore, Basade et al[37] have thoroughly reviewed the published trials concerning treatment of metastatic breast cancer with myeloablative high dose chemotherapy (HDCT) and autologous cell rescue. On the basis of trials published so far, HDCT has not proven to be superior to conventional chemotherapy for advanced breast cancer.

Breast nurse specialist

Specialist nurses have an established role in the management of breast cancer by offering counselling and emotional support. They are not usually involved in diagnosis. In an interesting study, it was shown that clinical nurse specialists could provide outpatient care.[38] Patients and their general practitioner had accepted the idea of being seen by specialist nurses. In addition, the nurses' clinical expertise compared favourably with that of other clinicians.

COLORECTAL CANCER

Hepatic perfusion index (HPI), which expresses the ratio of hepatic arterial to total liver blood flow, has been proposed as a possible method for detecting occult liver metastases in patients with colorectal cancer. This hypothesis was investigated in a prospective study which revealed that HPI predicts a poor outcome and may be useful in selection for adjuvant chemotherapy.[39]

Endothelin 1 (ET-1), a vasoconstrictor peptide, has been implicated as a tumour growth stimulator and an angiogenesis factor. Involvement of ET-1 in colorectal cancer was investigated by performing immunoelectron microscopy for ET-1 in colorectal liver metastases and normal liver, in addition to measuring ET-1 plasma levels by radioimmunoassay in patients with colorectal cancer, with and without liver metastases.[40] ET-1 was present in various cell types within colorectal liver metastases and raised levels were found in the plasma of patients with colorectal cancer. ET-1 may not only modulate tumour vascular tone but may also act on tumour growth and angiogenesis, both locally and systemically.

Early colorectal cancer

Accurate diagnosis, pre-operative and histopathological staging is crucial in the management of early colorectal adenocarcinoma. Detection of flat and depressed types of early lesions during colonoscopy requires awareness. Irregularity of the mucosal surface, pinkishness of the mucosa, fading of the mucosal colour, depressions and/or haemorrhagic spots are clues, which could help in early detection. Combined endoscopy and radiological examinations may detect 91% of sessile early colorectal carcinomas.[41]

Lymph node involvement varies from 0–15.4% in early colorectal cancer. Features which predict nodal metastases are tumour budding, the pattern of cancer growth in the submucosa, tumour differentiation, sessile configuration of the lesion, involvement of the rectum, and lymphatic and vascular invasion with cancer cells.

The treatment of early colorectal cancer is either surgical or endoscopic. Endoscopic polypectomy is suitable for small pedunculated lesions, with further treatment depending on histological findings, and this can be a definitive treatment for intramucosal cancer less than 3 cm in diameter. Radical surgical treatment is advisable for early colorectal cancer with suspected submucosal invasion. Indications for radical open surgery after polypectomy include involvement of the polypectomy margin with cancer, lymphatic invasion and inadequate tissue samples for accurate histological examination. Although the overall 5 year survival rate for patients with early colorectal cancers is 97.6%, lymph node invasion will reduce the rate to 56% and also increase the chance of cancer recurrence compared with node negative patients. Finally, several papers have reported a 5 year survival of 47–100% after excision by transanal endo-scopic microsurgery. This technique is also associated with a lower local recurrence rate than simple transanal excision.[41]

Surgical technique

The application of laparoscopic techniques to colorectal cancer resection has not gained universal acceptance because of the potential risk of cancer implantation in port sites. A prospective comparison of laparoscopic colorectal resection versus open resection in 54 consecutive patients has revealed significant early benefits for patients.[42] Adequate tumour clearance was achieved in the laparoscopic group, in addition no port-site or wound recurrence occurred after a median follow up of 28 months.

Weber et al[43] have reviewed the literature pertaining to local excision of distal rectal cancer, with and without adjuvant chemoradiotherapy. Different sphincter-sparing modalities were addressed. These include transanal endoscopic, trans-sphincteric, transcoccygeal, and trans-sacral approaches. The data do not support local excision as being superior or even equivalent to radical excision for invasive distal rectal carcinoma.

Primary resection and anastomosis of obstructed left-sided colorectal carcinoma is still debatable. Poon et al[44] analysed the safety and benefits of this approach in elderly patients. Some 57 elderly and 59 younger patients underwent emergency resection of an acutely obstructing left-sided colorectal carcinoma, with a primary anastomosis rate of 84% and 78%, respectively. Anastomotic leaks occurred in 6% of the elderly and 4% of younger patients. The hospital mortality rate was 9% and 5%, respectively. Therefore, emergency resection and primary anastomosis for left colorectal carcinoma can be performed safely in the elderly.

The results of resection of locoregional recurrence has been evaluated; 120 patients who underwent resection of colonic (56) or rectal (64) locoregional recurrence were analysed.[45] Sixty-nine curative resections, and nine synchronous hepatic resections were assessed. The hospital mortality rate was 7% and the morbidity rate was 40%. The overall 5 year survival rate was 27%. The results justify an attempt at resection whenever possible and long-term results might be improved with adjuvant therapy.

The development of new endoprostheses has enabled relief of large bowel obstruction, before operation. This might reduce morbidity and surgical death, in addition to avoiding the need for palliative colostomy. The major complication is colonic perforation, when dilatation of the stricture has to be performed before insertion of the metal stent.[46]

Adjuvant therapy

Two important clinical trials, which looked at the advantage of adjuvant chemotherapy after colorectal cancer surgical treatment, were recently published. The effect of adjuvant intraportal infusion of heparin and 5-fluorouracil (5-FU) on overall survival and disease-free survival in patients with resectable colon cancer were evaluated in a randomised controlled trial.[47] Some 235 patients were included, 79 patients in the control group, 72 patients infused intraportally with heparin (5000 IU daily for 7 consecutive days) and 84 patients who were given intraportal heparin and 5-FU (500 mg/m² daily for 7 consecutive days). No differences were observed between the control group and treatment groups for postoperative complications and length of hospitalisation. After a median 9 years of follow-up and based on all randomised patients, the effect of treatment was not statistically significant. It was also concluded that intraportal 5-FU infusion is safe and has a tolerable toxicity, but it was not considered standard therapy for patients with resectable colon cancer.

Irinotecan is a topoisomerase I inhibitor that blocks DNA replication of the enzyme, leading to multiple single-strand DNA breaks, which eventually blocks cell division. The overall benefits of this agent have been evaluated in a randomised clinical trial.[48] Patients with metastatic colorectal cancer, in whom 6 months' treatment with 5-FU had failed to stop disease progression, were randomly treated with either 300–350 mg/m^2 irinotecan every 3 weeks with supportive care or supportive care only in a 2:1 ratio (189:90, respectively). With a median follow-up of 13 months, overall survival was significantly higher in the irinotecan group. It was, therefore, confirmed that despite the side effects of treatment, patients who have metastatic colorectal cancer, and for whom 5-FU has failed, have a longer survival, fewer tumour-related symptoms, and a better quality of life when treated with irinotecan than when treated with supportive care alone. Thus, irinotecan can be recommended as a second line treatment.

The effect of adjuvant radiotherapy on local recurrence and survival after rectal cancer resection was reviewed in depth by Heriot et al.[49] It was revealed that pre-operative radiotherapy is more effective in reducing local recurrence than postoperative radiotherapy. However, postoperative chemoradiotherapy is associated with a survival benefit, although it has high toxicity. In addition, systemically or intraportally administered fluorouracil-containing chemotherapy can produce a survival advantage in Dukes' C colonic cancer. There was no evidence to suggest such benefit with rectal cancers.

Finally, Maxwell-Armstrong et al[50] have highlighted the exciting idea of colorectal cancer vaccination. Vaccines have been developed that stimulate the immune system to target colorectal 17-1A, 791 Tgb 72 and carcinoembryonic antigens. A number of approaches are currently being evaluated, these include anti-idiotypic antibody immunisation, DNA vaccines, mucin and heat shock protein-based vaccines, in addition to oncogenes and viral vectors.

ANAL PROBLEMS

ANAL FISTULA

Surgical management of high anal fistula by cutting seton and the two-stage seton fistulotomy (TSSF) were studied by Garc'ia-Aguilar et al.[51] 59 patients were treated with cutting seton or TSSF over a 5 year period and no differences in the rate of recurrence of fistula between the groups was found. Both techniques were equally effective in eradicating the fistula, and were associated with a similar rate of incontinence. In another study, a modified seton technique, in which a rubber band was pulled through the fistula track and tightened around the external sphincter by a thread, has been described.[52] Patient tolerance and anal continence were satisfactory.

Robertson et al[53] treated 23 anal fistulas in 20 patients with cutaneous advancement flap after suture closure of the internal opening and adequate drainage of the external opening. In the non-inflammatory bowel disease group, complete healing of all wounds occurred in 11 of 14 patients at an average of 6.5 weeks (average follow-up 18 months). Complications included donor site separation in two patients and minor incontinence of flatus in one patient. In the inflammatory bowel disease group, five fistulas healed, two failed, and one patient developed a new fistula during an average follow-up of 16 months. The performance of stricturectomy in conjunction with circumferential rectal sleeve advancement for patients who have a rectovaginal fistula arising from an anorectal Crohn's stricture provides a good repair in addition to correction of the stricture and maintains continence.[54]

A total of 103 consecutive patients, with uncomplicated intersphincteric or trans-sphincteric fistula *in ano*, were randomised to have either the wounds left open or wound edges marsupialized to the fistula tract with interrupted absorbable sutures.[55] Hospitalisation and complication rates were the same in both groups. Anal fistulotomy wounds healed faster after marsupialization, and anal squeeze pressures were better preserved. This may improve anal continence.

ANAL FISSURE

Chronic anal fissure has traditionally been treated by surgery. In a recent paper, alternative forms of treatment for chronic anal fissure were retrospectively assessed.[56] Manual dilatation of the anus, lateral internal sphincterotomy and topical GTN ointment, were first choice. According to this assessment, lateral internal sphincterotomy has replaced anal digital dilatation as a primary treatment, and GTN cream has increasingly been offered as a first line of treatment over the last 12 months. Furthermore, the use of peri-operative endo-anal ultrasound allowed identification of high risk patients who may develop post-sphincterotomy incontinence. An anal advancement flap has been used as an alternative surgical approach for these patients.

HAEMORRHOIDS

Haemorrhoidectomy is usually an in-patient procedure because patients and doctors worry about postoperative pain. Day case haemorrhoidectomy (DCH) is possible, particularly if patient anxiety is addressed and postoperative pain and bowel function are treated. The possibility of secondary infection as a cause of post-haemorrhoidectomy pain was studied.[57] Forty consecutive patients admitted for DCH were randomly treated with either metronidazole 400 mg or placebo 3 times daily, both for 7 days. All patients received lactulose for 2 days before surgery and for 2 weeks after. Diathermy DCH was performed without pedicle ligation, and a diclofenac suppository was administered at the end of the procedure. Patients were discharged on the same day with diclofenac, 0.2% glyceryl trinitrate ointment and lactulose. This study demonstrates that prophylactic metronidazole in DCH suppresses postoperative pain and increases patient satisfaction.

INFLAMMATORY BOWEL DISEASE

Ileal pouch-anal anastomosis for chronic ulcerative colitis was first described in 1978 and has become a well established procedure. Postoperative complications and functional outcome after hand-sewn single J-shaped pouch were prospectively assessed in 1,310 patients.[58] Increased experience reduces pouch-related complications. The functional results in term of mean number of daily stools and incontinence, remains steady with time, although pouch failure increases.

Intra-abdominal and pelvic abscesses occur in 10–30% of patients with Crohn's disease due to a localised perforation resulting in an abscess cavity communicating with the bowel lumen. The management and outcome of 36 patients with such abscesses, of whom 15 were considered for initial percutaneous drainage, were reviewed by Jawhari et al.[59] Crohn's intra-abdominal abscesses are associated with a high morbidity rate and percutaneous drainage can be performed in selected cases, without adding to the complications.

HEPATOBILIARY SURGERY

LIVER

Traumatic liver injury

Non-operative management is the treatment of choice in over 50% of adult patients with blunt liver injury. Carrillo et al[60] reviewed the criteria for non-operative management and was shown to be safe in haemodynamically stable patients in 50–80% of cases. Computed tomography (CT) of the abdomen is extremely useful to document the extent of the damage and the presence of associated injuries, but it is not possible, based on CT alone, to predict failure. Hence, careful physiological monitoring in selected patients is indicated to avoid catastrophic complications.

Liver abscess

Management of liver abscesses with intravenous antibiotics and radiologically controlled percutaneous drainage is generally acceptable. However, not all abscesses are treated successfully in this way, and some may require surgical drainage. Laparoscopic drainage of liver abscesses, in combination with systemic antibiotics has been reported a safe and viable alternative following failed medical or percutaneous treatment.[61] There were no intra-operative or postoperative complications.

Liver cysts

Diez et al[62] successfully treated both solitary and multiple liver cysts by a laparoscopic approach, which resulted in minimal surgical trauma and shorter hospital stay.

Percutaneous drainage of hepatic hydatid cysts has been compared with traditional surgical cystectomy.[63] In 50 patients randomly allocated to either percutaneous drainage or open cystectomy, percutaneous drainage combined with albendazole was an effective and safe alternative to surgery and required a shorter hospital stay.

Liver tumour

In two studies, the volume of blood loss following liver resection was correlated with the CVP. Lowering the pressure in the IVC to less than 5 cm H_2O is the key to reducing blood loss during liver surgery.[64,65]

Percutaneous cryosurgical liver tumour ablation has been described for patients with inadequately resected liver metastases from colorectal cancer and local disease control was considerably improved by cryoablation.[66,67]

GALLBLADDER DISEASE

Laparoscopic cholecystectomy has been deemed a safe procedure in numerous clinical trials, regardless of the known increased risk of bile duct injury. However, the consequences and incidence of less well-known complications are still being addressed. In a randomised trial, early laparoscopic cholecystectomy was compared with delayed laparoscopic cholecystectomy.[68] There was no significant difference in conversion rate, postoperative analgesia requirement or complications. It was felt that early laparoscopic cholecystectomy is safe and feasible for acute cholecystitis.

Complications of laparoscopic cholecystectomy

The management and outcome of bile leaks and bile duct strictures following the introduction of laparoscopic cholecystectomy was reviewed in an interesting paper.[69] Cystic stump or segment V leaks were treated successfully by endoscopic stenting. Roux loop biliary reconstruction was carried out to repair CHD strictures and bile duct trans-sections. All had normal liver function test results at a median follow-up of 30 months. Patients with partial duct injuries, repaired at initial surgery, required no further intervention.

Endoscopic sphincterotomy, stent placement, or sphincterotomy with stent are effective in healing biliary leaks after laparoscopic cholecystectomy with good patient tolerance.[70]

Gall stone spillage

A retrospective study of more than ten thousand laparoscopic cholecystectomies has revealed that 6% of patients had gallstone leakage, and 0.08% developed subsequent abscesses.[71] The infected gallstones have been reported to have traversed the diaphragm, migrated into the lung parenchyma, and obstructed a segmental bronchus, causing pneumonia. Subphrenic abscess around spilled gallstones can form a thoracic empyema.[72] Treatment involves retrieval of the stones, drainage of the pleuroperitoneal abscess and intravenous antibiotics. A chronic sub-hepatic abscess around a lost intraperitoneally retained stone has lead to obstructive cholangitis.[73]

Operative cholangiography

In a prospective audit of biliary injury, operative cholangiography was not found to be a prerequisite for the safe performance of laparoscopic cholecystectomy.[74] All biliary injuries were recorded. Meticulous dissection proved to be a reliable safeguard against injury to the right hepatic, common hepatic and common bile ducts. However, four accessory ducts were sacrificed and localised injury to the common hepatic or common bile duct occurred in three patients. According to the above findings, these injuries would not have been prevented by operative cholangiography. In another study, however, 85% of bile duct injuries occurred when an intra-operative cholangiography was not performed.[75]

Common bile duct

The accuracy of magnetic resonance cholangiography (MRC) to detect choledocholithiasis in selected patients before laparoscopic cholecystectomy has been evaluated.[76] It proved to be a simple non-invasive method for pre-operative screening of common bile duct stones in high risk patients and can reduce the need for ERCP or intra-operative cholangiography in identifying asymptomatic CBD stones.[77]

The indications for endoscopic sphincterotomy (ES) have been extended to young patients with choledocholithiasis with long-term follow-up.[78] Approximately 10% of patients developed late complications.

Common bile duct stones can be removed in a large proportion of patients undergoing laparoscopic cholecystectomy, either by a laparoscopic transcystic technique or through a laparoscopic choledochotomy.[79]

PANCREATIC DISEASE

PANCREATITIS

Early detection of infected pancreatic necrosis has a major impact on management and outcome in acute pancreatitis. Rau et al[80] evaluated ultrasonographically guided fine-needle aspiration cytology in necrotizing pancreatitis. It is fast and reliable and recommended for all patients with necrotizing pancreatitis in which the systemic inflammatory response syndrome persists beyond the first week following onset of symptoms.

Endoscopic sphincterotomy alone, or followed by cholecystectomy, are options in patients with gallstone pancreatitis. Ninety-six patients (median age 74 years, range 30–93 years) with gallstone pancreatitis had ERC and were followed for a median of 84 months (range 33–168 months). Endoscopic sphincterotomy, but not interval cholecystectomy, reduced the overall incidence of recurrent pancreatitis. Some 31% of the patients required cholecystectomy, suggesting that routine cholecystectomy should be considered in fit patients following ES after acute pancreatitis.[81]

Acute biliary pancreatitis necessitates urgent diagnosis and treatment of common bile duct (CBD) stones. The roles of urgent endoscopic ultrasono-graphy (EUS) and endoscopic retrograde cholangiopancreatography (ERCP) in the management of biliary pancreatitis were prospectively studied.[82] EUS, an accurate and less invasive modality, may limit ERCP to therapeutic use in biliary pancreatitis. EUS is recommended if ultrasonography and CT have failed to detect CBD stones.

The complications of diagnostic and therapeutic ERCP have been reported[83] in 2,769 consecutive patients in 9 centres over a 2 year period; 111 major complications (4.0%) were recorded including moderate/severe pancreatitis (1.3%), cholangitis (0.87%), haemorrhage (0.76%) and duodenal perforation (0.58%). Amongst 942 diagnostic ERCP, there were 13 major complications (1.38%) and 2 deaths (0.21%); whereas among 1,827 therapeutic ERCP there were 98 major complications (5.4%) and 9 deaths (0.49%). The difference in the incidence of complications between diagnostic and therapeutic ERCP was statistically significant.

What's new in general surgery – a review of the journals

PANCREATIC TUMOURS

Isolated hypoxic perfusion with mitomycin C in patients with unresectable or recurrent pancreatic cancer did not show any benefit in tumour response and median survival.[84]

Pancreatic cancer resection is said to be a high risk procedure in patients over 70 years old. However, operative outcome and survival in 33 patients aged 70 years or more compared with findings in 85 younger patients showed no significant difference in resectability nor any difference in mortality or overall morbidity.[85] Accordingly, patients aged 70 years or more can benefit from pancreatic cancer resection similarly to younger patients.

Cystic tumours of the pancreas

Of all cystic tumours, 90% are epithelial tumours, either benign cystadenomas (serous or mucinous) or malignant cystadenocarcinomas. Histological examination after pancreatic resection is the only way to differentiate between benign and malignant mucinous cystic lesions. Mucinous cystadenomas should be resected completely with more than a 50% 5 year survival rate. Adjuvant therapy should be considered for aneuploid tumours. Finally, pseudopapillary solid cystic tumour should be resected completely because of potential malignancy.[86]

THYROID AND PARATHYROID DISEASE

Controversy continues regarding the optimal extent of thyroid resection in patients with papillary thyroid carcinoma who are at minimal risk of cause-specific mortality (CSM). The outcome in patients undergoing either unilateral lobectomy or total thyroidectomy was evaluated after a mean follow-up of 18 years.[87] Unilateral lobectomy was not associated with higher CSM rates, but was associated with a significantly higher risk of locoregional recurrence. It was also reported that, at 5 years, there were no differences in survival between lobectomy or total thyroidectomy for any subgroup with papillary or follicular carcinoma.[88]

The 10 year overall survival rates for US patients with papillary, follicular, Hurthle cell, medullary, and undifferentiated anaplastic carcinoma were 93%, 85%, 76%, 75%, and 14%, respectively. Total thyroidectomy, with and without lymph node sampling, represent the major surgical treatment for papillary and follicular neoplasms. Approximately 38% of such patients received adjuvant iodine-131 ablation therapy. Sato et al[89] suggested that the presence of histologically confirmed lymph node metastases is not an important prognostic factor in patients with differentiated thyroid carcinoma followed for 2–27 years (median, 7 years). It was shown that the only statistically significant adverse prognostic factors were age > 45 years, distant metastases and TNM stage.

Postoperative measurements of serum thyroglobulin (Tg) are currently used as a marker of recurrent disease or distant metastases in the follow-up of patients with differentiated thyroid cancer. To investigate whether Tg levels differ in benign and malignant follicular and Hurthle cell neoplasms, pre-operative serum Tg measurements were performed.[90] Tg concentration was measured in addition to the standard pre-operative tests (fine-needle aspiration biopsy, ultrasonography, ^{99m}Tc scanning and hormonal profile). Pre-operative serum Tg measurements might be an important additional diagnostic tool in patients with thyroid tumours.

MINIMALLY INVASIVE RADIO-GUIDED PARATHYROIDECTOMY

Operations for hyperparathyroidism (HPT) in a previously operated neck present a significant challenge and carry much higher morbidity rates than first-time operations. Minimally invasive radio-guided parathyroidectomy (MIRP) has been reported as an efficient procedure in patients who have undergone previous neck exploration for parathyroid or thyroid disease.[91] Eighteen patients underwent MIRP under local anaesthesia as outpatients; in addition 3 MIRPs were done under general anaesthesia. Average operative time was 44 min, average incision length was 3.0 ± 0.2 cm. Nineteen of the procedures were completed without frozen section. There were no complications.

FINE NEEDLE ASPIRATION CYTOLOGY

Giovagnoli et al[92] have again identified the limitations of FNA to differentiate between follicular adenomas from well-differentiated follicular carcinomas. Nevertheless, FNA with ultrasonographic support has been accepted as a guide in selecting patients who need surgery, and could be useful for detecting non palpable thyroid nodules larger than 10 mm.[93] In another study, the predictive value of pre-operative fine-needle aspiration on surgical decision making was evaluated in comparison to intra-operative frozen section.[94] There was no evidence to suggest that intra-operative frozen section adds much to intra-operative decision making in patients with thyroid cancer.

MISCELLANEOUS CONDITIONS

MALIGNANT ASCITES

Malignant ascites is associated with a very poor prognosis. Matrix metalloproteinases (MMP) are enzymes, shown to be important in tumour invasion and metastasis. In a variety of cancers, including colorectal, gastric, and breast cancer, a MMP inhibitor (basimatastat) has been evaluated clinically and shown to be useful in controlling ascites.[95] It is well absorbed intraperitoneally and caused few side effects.

INGUINAL HERNIA REPAIR

Wellwood et al[96] compared tension free open mesh hernioplasty under local anaesthetic with transabdominal preperitoneal laparoscopic hernia repair under general anaesthetic. Although the laparoscopic approach was more expensive in comparison to open repair, it was considered to have short-term clinical advantages especially on the early return to normal activity in addition to greater patient satisfaction. Instillation of local anaesthetic into the preperitoneal space resulted in no significant effect on postoperative pain relief requirement following laparoscopic hernia repair.[97]

MELANOMA

The use of elective regional node dissection in patients with cutaneous melanoma without clinical evidence of metastatic spread is debatable. In patients with 1.5 mm or more thickness, and without clinical evidence of regional node and distant metastases, node dissection results in an increased survival in patients with node metastases only.[98] Therefore, sentinel node biopsy may become valuable to identify patients with occult node metastases, who could then undergo complete node dissection.

NEW MODALITIES FOR CONTROL OF CANCER

Exciting reports have featured the possible benefit of anti-angiogenesis drugs and ultrasonic bloodless surgery in cancer treatment.

The growth of tumours depends on angiogenesis. Therefore, the interest in the development of drugs to inhibit tumour angiogenesis is growing. One of these anti-angiogenesis agents is angiostatin, produced by the metallo-proteinase stromelysin I. Administration of angiostatin inhibits growth of primary tumours and metastases by prevention of blood vessel formation and causes death of tumour cells by apoptosis. Endostatin is another angiogenesis inhibitor, which has caused almost complete regression of tumours. Combination of angiostatin and endostatin may be more effective and could offer a cure for cancer in the future.[99]

High intensity focused ultrasound (HIFU) is a new ultrasound technology which could revolutionise our surgical practice. HIFU uses transducers that generate energies 10,000 times more powerful than those used in diagnostic ultrasound. In a phase I trial, 23 patients with primary prostate, kidney tumours, or with liver metastases were treated.[100] Treatment was well tolerated without anaesthesia. The HIFU technique might be superior to surgical cautery as it can cauterise tissue deep within an organ, which can then be cut away with minimal bleeding.

References

1. Demedts I, Tack J. Chest pain of esophageal origin. Curr Opin Gastroenterol 1998; 14: 340–344.
2. Martinez de Haro L, Ortiz A, Parrilla P et al. Clinical features and investigations in patients with columnar-lined oesophagus. Br J Surg 1998; 85: 1150–1152.
3. Di Stefano A, Russello D N A, Bloch P. Gastro-oesophageal reflux. Comparison of laparoscopic and open procedures. Eighty cases and literature review. Chirurgia 1998; 11: 71–75.
4. Anvari M, Allen C. Laparoscopic Nissen fundoplication two-year comprehensive follow-up of a technique of minimal paraesophageal dissection. Ann Surg 1998; 227: 25–32.
5. Krasna M J. Advances in staging of esophageal carcinoma. Chest 1998; 113: 107S–111S.

6. Romijn M G, Van Overhagen H, Bilgen E J S et al. Laparoscopy and laparoscopic ultrasonography in staging of oesophageal and cardial carcinoma. Br J Surg 1998; 85: 1010–1012.

7. Riedel M, Hauck R W, Stein H J et al. Preoperative bronchoscopic assessment of airway invasion by esophageal cancer: a prospective study. Chest 1998; 113: 687–695.

8. Sykes A J, Burt P A, Slevin N J et al. Radical radiotherapy for carcinoma of the oesophagus: an effective alternative to surgery. Radiother Oncol 1998; 48: 15–21.

9. Nishihira T, Hirayama K, Mori S A. Prospective randomized trial of extended cervical and superior mediastinal lymphadenectomy for carcinoma of the thoracic esophagus. Am J Surg 1998; 175: 47–51.

10. Craig S R, Adam D J, Peng L Y et al. Effect of blood transfusion on survival after esophagogastrectomy for carcinoma. Ann Thorac Surg 1998; 66: 356–361.

11. Chow L W C, Gertsch P, Poon R T P. Risk factor for rebleeding and death from peptic ulcer in the very elderly. Br J Surg 1998; 85, 121–124.

12. Zimmer T, Rucktaschel F, Stolzel U et al. Endoscopic sclerotherapy with fibrin glue as compared with polidocanol to prevent early esophageal variceal rebleeding. J Hepatol 1998; 28: 292–297.

13. Sung J J Y, Chung S C S. The use of a detachable mini-loop for the treatment of esophageal varices. Gastrointest Endosc 1998; 47: 178–181.

14. Sanchez Bueno F, Garcia-Marcilla J A, Perez-Flores D et al. Prognostic factors in a series of 297 patients with gastric adenocarcinoma undergoing surgical resection. Br J Surg 1998; 85: 255–260.

15. Cascinu S, Labianca R, Graziano F et al. Intensive weekly chemotherapy for locally advanced gastric cancer using 5-fluorouracil, cisplatin, epidoxorubicin, 6S-leucovorin, glutathione and filgrastim: a report from the Italian Group for the Study of Digestive Tract Cancer (GISCAD). Br J Cancer 1998; 78: 390–393.

16. Helicobacter pylori and gastric cancer. Drug Ther Bull 1998, 36: 57–59.

17. Furukawa H, Hiratsuka M, Imaoka S et al. Limited surgery for early gastric cancer in cardia. Ann Surg Oncol 1998; 5: 338–341.

18. Roukos D H, Lorenz M, Encke A. Evidence of survival benefit of extended (D2) lymphadenectomy in western patients with gastric cancer based on a new concept: a prospective long-term follow-up study. Surgery 1998; 123: 573–578.

19. Degiuli M, Sasako M, Ponti A et al. Morbidity and mortality after D2 gastrectomy for gastric cancer: results of the Italian Gastric Cancer Study Group prospective multicenter surgical study. J Clin Oncol 1998; 16: 1490–1493.

20. Schepotin I B, Chorny V A, Nauta R J et al. Extended surgical resection in T4 gastric cancer. Am J Surg 1998; 175: 123–126.

21. Ikeda M, Ueda T, Shiba T. Reconstruction after total gastrectomy by the interposition of a double jejunal pouch using a double stapling technique. Br J Surg 1998; 85: 398–402.

22. Andersen B L, Farrar W B, Golden-Kreutz D et al. Stress and immune responses after surgical treatment for regional breast cancer. J Natl Cancer Inst 1998; 90: 30–36.

23. Saad Z, Bramwell V H C, Wilson S M et al. Expression of genes that contribute to proliferative and metastatic ability in breast cancer resected during various menstrual phases. Lancet 1998; 351: 1170–1173.

24. Colditz G A. Relationship between estrogen levels, use of hormone replacement therapy, and breast cancer. J Natl Cancer Inst 1998; 90: 814–823.

25. Verhoog L C, Brekelmans C T M, Seynaeve C et al. Survival and tumour characteristics of breast cancer patients with germline mutations of BRCA1. Lancet 1998; 351: 316.

26. Powles T, Eeles R, Ashley S et al. Interim analysis of the incidence of breast cancer in the Royal Marsden Hospital tamoxifen randomised chemoprevention trial. Lancet 1998; 352: 98–101.

27. Veronesi U, Maisonneuve P, Costa A et al. Prevention of breast cancer with tamoxifen: preliminary findings from the Italian randomised trial among hysterectomised women. Italian Tamoxifen Prevention Study. Lancet 1998; 352: 93–97.

28. Schroen A M, Wobbes T, van der Sluis R F. Infiltrating lobular carcinoma of the breast detected by screening. Br J Surg 1998; 85: 390–392.

29. Markandoo P, Smith P, Chaudary M A et al. Preservation of pectoralis minor in axillary clearance for breast cancer. Br J Surg 1998; 85: 1547–1548.

What's new in general surgery – a review of the journals

Recent Advances in Surgery 23

30. Abdullah T I, Iddon J, Barr L et al. Prospective randomized controlled trial of preservation of the intercostobrachial nerve during axillary node clearance for breast cancer. Br J Surg 1998; 85: 1443–1445.

31. Beck N E, Bradburn M J, Vincenti A C et al. Detection of residual disease following breast-conserving surgery. Br J Surg 1998; 85: 1273–1276.

32. Vyas J J, Chinoy R F, Vaidya J S. Prediction of nipple and areola involvement in breast cancer. Eur J Surg Oncol 1998; 24: 15–16.

33. McIntosh S A, Purushotham A D. Lymphatic mapping and sentinel node biopsy in breast cancer. Br J Surg 1998; 85: 1347–1356.

34. Flett M M, Going J J, Stanton P D et al. Sentinel node localization in patients with breast cancer. Br J Surg 1998; 85: 991–993.

35. Kapteijn B A E, Nieweg O E, Petersen J L et al. Identification and biopsy of the sentinel lymph node in breast cancer. Eur J Surg Oncol 1998; 24: 427–430.

36. Rodenhuis S, Richel D J, van der Wall E et al. Randomised trial of high-dose chemotherapy and haemopoietic progenitor-cell support in operable breast cancer with extensive axillary lymph-node involvement. Lancet 1998; 352: 515–521.

37. Basade M M, Gulati S C. High-dose chemotherapy in metastatic breast cancer. Lancet 1998; 351: 386–387.

38. Garvican L, Grimsey E, Littlejohns P et al. Satisfaction with clinical nurse specialists in a breast care clinic: questionnaire survey. BMJ 1998: 316: 976–977.

39. Warren H W, Gallagher H, Hemingway D M. Prospective assessment of the hepatic perfusion index in patients with colorectal cancer. Br J Surg 1998; 85: 1708–1721.

40. Shankar A, Loizidou M, Aliev G et al. Raised endothelin 1 levels in patients with colorectal liver metastases. Br J Surg 1998; 85: 502–506.

41. Mainprize K S, Mortensen N J McC, Warren B F Early colorectal cancer: recognition, classification and treatment. Br J Surg 1998; 85: 469–476.

42. Psaila J, Bulley S H, Ewings P. Outcome following laparoscopic resection for colorectal cancer. Br J Surg 1998; 85: 662–664.

43. Weber T K, Petrelli N J. Local excision for rectal cancer: an uncertain future. Oncology 1998; 12: 933–947.

44. Poon R T, Law W L, Chu K W. Emergency resection and primary anastomosis for left-sided obstructing colorectal carcinoma in the elderly. Br J Surg 1998; 85: 1539–1542.

45. Delpero J R, Pol B, Le Treut Y P. Surgical resection of locally recurrent colorectal adenocarcinoma. Br J Surg 1998; 85: 372–376.

46. Akle C A. Endoprostheses for colonic strictures. Br J Surg 1998; 85: 310–314.

47. Nitti D, Wils J, Sahmoud T et al. Final results of a phase III clinical trial on adjuvant intraportal infusion with heparin and 5-fluorouracil (5-FU) in resectable colon cancer. Eur J Cancer 1997; 33: 1209–1215.

48. Cunningham D, Pyrhonen S, James U D et al. Randomised trial of irinotecan plus supportive care versus supportive care alone after fluorouracil failure for patients with metastatic colorectal cancer. Lancet 1998; 352: 1413–1418.

49. Heriot A G, Kumar D. Adjuvant therapy for resectable rectal and colonic cancer. Br J Surg 1998; 85: 300–309.

50. Maxwell-Armstrong C A, Durrant L G, Scholefield J H. Colorectal cancer vaccines. Br J Surg 1998; 85: 149–154.

51. Garc'ia-Aguilar J, Belmonte C, Wong D W et al. Cutting seton versus two-stage seton fistulotomy in the surgical management of high anal fistula. Br J Surg 1998; 85: 243–245.

52. Dziki A; Bartos M. Seton treatment of anal fistula: experience with a new modification. Eur J Surg 1998; 164: 543–548.

53. Robertson W G; Mangione J S. Cutaneous advancement flap closure: alternative method for treatment of complicated anal fistulas. Dis Colon Rectum 1998; 41: 884–886.

54. Simmang C L, Lacey S W; Huber Jr P J. Rectal sleeve advancement: repair of rectovaginal fistula associated with anorectal stricture in Crohn's disease. Dis Colon Rectum 1998; 41: 787–789.

55. Ho Y H, Tan M, Leong A F et al. Marsupialization of fistulotomy wounds improves healing: a randomized controlled trial. Br J Surg 1998; 85: 105–107.

56. Farouk R, Duthie G S, Gunn J. Changing patterns of treatment for chronic anal fissure. Ann R Coll Surg Engl 1998; 80: 194–196.

57. Carapeti E A, Kamm M A, McDonald P J et al. Double-blind randomised controlled trial of effect of metronidazole on pain after day-case haemorrhoidectomy. Lancet 1998; 351; 169–172.

58. Meagher A P, Farouk R. Dozois R R J. Ileal pouch-anal anastomosis for chronic ulcerative colitis: complications and long-term outcome in 1310 patients. Br J Surg 1998; 85: 800–803.

59. Jawhari A, Kamm M A, Ong C. Intra-abdominal and pelvic abscess in Crohn's disease: results of non-invasive and surgical management. Br J Surg 1998; 85: 367–371.

60. Carrillo E H, Platz A, Miller F B et al. Non-operative management of blunt hepatic trauma. Br J Surg 1998; 85: 461–468.

61. Tay K H, Ravintharan T, Hoe M N et al. Laparoscopic drainage of liver abscesses. Br J Surg 1998; 85: 330–332.

62. Diez J, Decoud J, Gutierrez L et al. Laparoscopic treatment of symptomatic cysts of the liver. Br J Surg 1998; 85: 25–27.

63. Khuroo M S, Wani N A, Javid G et al. Percutaneous drainage compared with surgery for hepatic hydatid cysts. N Engl J Med 1997; 337: 881–887.

64. Johnson M, Mannar R, Wu A V O. Correlation between blood loss and inferior vena caval pressure during liver resection. Br J Surg 1998; 85: 188–190.

65. Jones R McL, Moulton C E, Hardy K J. Central venous pressure and its effect on blood loss during liver resection Br J Surg 1998; 85: 1058–1060.

66. Adam R, Majno P, Castaing D. Treatment of irresectable liver tumours by percutaneous cryosurgery. Br J Surg 1998; 85: 1493–1494.

67. Dwerryhouse S J, Seifert J K, McCall J L. Hepatic resection with cryotherapy to involved or inadequate resection margin (edge freeze) for metastases from colorectal cancer. Br J Surg 1998; 85: 185–187.

68. Lai P B S, Kwong K H, Leung K L et al. Randomized trial of early versus delayed laparoscopic cholecystectomy for acute cholecystitis. Br J Surg 1998; 85: 764–767.

69. Doctor N, Dooley J S. Dick R et al. Multidisciplinary approach to biliary complications of laparoscopic cholecystectomy. Br J Surg 1998; 85: 627–632.

70. Ryan M E, Geenen J E, Lehman G A et al. Endoscopic intervention for biliary leaks after laparoscopic cholecystectomy: a multicenter review. Gastrointest Endosc 1998; 47: 261–266.

71. Schafer M, Suter C, Klaiber Ch et al. Spilled gallstones after laparoscopic cholecystectomy: a relevant problem? A retrospective analysis of 10,174 laparoscopic cholecystectomies. Surg Endosc 1998; 12: 305–309.

72. Kelty C J. Thorpe J A C. Empyema due to spilled stones during laparoscopic cholecystectomy. Eur J Cardiothorac Surg 1998; 13: 107–108.

73. Petit F, Vons C, Tahrat M et al. Jaundice following laparoscopic cholecystectomy: an unusual complication of spilled stones. Surg Endosc 1998; 12: 450–451.

74. Wright K D, Wellwood J M. Bile duct injury during laparoscopic cholecystectomy without operative cholangiography. Br J Surg 1998; 85: 191–194.

75. Torkington J, Chalmers R T A, Pereira J. Laparoscopic cholecystectomy, bile duct injury and the British and Irish surgeon. Ann R Coll Surg Engl 1998; 80: 119–121.

76. Dwerryhouse S J, Brown E, Vipond M N. Prospective evaluation of magnetic resonance cholangiography to detect common bile duct stones before laparoscopic cholecystectomy. Br J Surg 1998; 85: 1364–1366.

77. Musella M, Barbalace G, Capparelli G. Magnetic resonance imaging in evaluation of the common bile duct. Br J Surg 1998; 85: 16–19.

78. Sugiyama M, Atomi Y. Follow-up of more than 10 years after endoscopic sphincterotomy for choledocholithiasis in young patients. Br J Surg 1998; 85: 917–921.

79. Arvidsson D N A, Berggren U, Haglund U. Laparoscopic common bile duct exploration. Eur J Surg 1998; 164: 369–375.

80. Rau B, Pralle U, Mayer J M et al. Role of ultrasonographically guided fine-needle aspiration cytology in the diagnosis of infected pancreatic necrosis. Br J Surg 1998; 85: 179–184.

81. Hammarstrom L E, Stridbeck H, Ihse I. Effect of endoscopic sphincterotomy and interval cholecystectomy on late outcome after gallstone pancreatitis. Br J Surg 1998; 85: 333–336.

82. Sugiyama M, Atomi Y. Acute biliary pancreatitis: the roles of endoscopic ultrasonography and endoscopic retrograde cholangiopancreatography. Surgery 1998; 124: 14–21.

83. Loperfido S, Angelini G, Benedetti G et al. Major early complications from diagnostic and therapeutic ERCP: a prospective multicenter study. Gastrointest Endosc 1998; 48: 1–10.

84. Lorenz M, Petrowsky S, Heinrich S et al. Isolated hypoxic perfusion with mitomycin C in patients with advanced pancreatic cancer. Eur J. Surg Oncol 1998; 24: 542–547.

85. Dicarlo V, Balzano G, Zerbi A. Pancreatic cancer resection in elderly patients. Br J Surg 1998; 85: 607–610.

86. Le Borgne J. Cystic tumours of the pancreas. Br J Surg 1998; 85: 577–579.

87. Hay I D, Grant C S, Bergstrahl E J. Unilateral total lobectomy: is it sufficient surgical treatment for patients with AMES low-risk papillary thyroid carcinoma?. Surgery 1998; 124: 958–964.

88. Hundahl S A, Fleming I D, Fremgen A M et al. A National Cancer Data Base report on 53,856 cases of thyroid carcinoma treated in the U.S., 1985–1995. Cancer 1998; 83: 2638–2648.

89. Sato N, Oyamatsu M, Koyama Y. Do the level of nodal disease according to the TNM classification and the number of involved cervical nodes reflect prognosis in patients with differentiated carcinoma of the thyroid gland?. J Surg Oncol 1998; 69: 151–155.

90. Hocevar M, Auersperg M. Role of serum thyroglobulin in the pre-operative evaluation of follicular thyroid tumours. Eur J Surg Oncol 1998; 24: 553–557.

91. Norman J, Denham D. Minimally invasive radioguided parathyroidectomy in the reoperative neck. Surgery 1998; 124:1088–1092.

92. Giovagnoli M R, Pisani T, Drusco A. Fine needle aspiration biopsy in the preoperative management of patients with thyroid nodules. Anticancer Res 1998; 18: 3741–3745.

93. Hagag P, Strauss S, Weiss M. Role of ultrasound-guided fine-needle aspiration biopsy in evaluation of nonpalpable thyroid nodules. Thyroid 1998; 8: 989–995.

94. Boyd L A, Earnhardt R C, Dunn J T. Preoperative evaluation and predictive value of fine-needle aspiration and frozen section of thyroid nodules. J Am Coll Surg 1998; 187: 494–502.

95. Parsons S L, Watson S A, Steele R J. Phase I/II trial of batimastat, a matrix metalloproteinase inhibitor, in patients with malignant ascites. Eur J Surg Oncol 1998; 23: 526–531.

96. Wellwood J, Sculpher M J, Stoker D et al. Randomised controlled trial of laparoscopic versus open mesh repair for inguinal hernia: outcome and cost. BMJ 1998; 317: 103–110.

97. Deans G T, Wilson M S, Brough W A. Controlled trial of preperitoneal local anaesthetic for reducing pain following hernia repair. Br J Surg 1998; 85: 1013–1014.

98. Cascinelli N, Morabito A, Santinami M et al. Immediate or delayed dissection of regional nodes in patients with melanoma of the trunk: a randomised trial. WHO Melanoma Programme. Lancet 1998; 351: 793–796.

99. Harris A L. Are angiostatin and endostatin cures for cancer?. Lancet 1998; 351: 1598–1599.

100. McCarthy M. Bloodless surgery: ultrasound cleans up operations. Lancet 1998; 352: 1450.

Index

V

Varicose veins, 125–32
    and deep vein reflux, 126
    and drug treatment, 137
    perforating veins, 127
    recurrent, 132–3
    sapheno-femoral junction (SFJ), 127
    sapheno-popliteal junction (SPJ), 127
    small, management, 131–2
    stripper wire, 128
    surgical treatments, 126–31
Vascular surgery
    and evidence-based medicine, 30–1
    review, 23–32
Veins
    disease, modern approaches, 125–40
    medial calf perforation, ligation, 135

    ulceration, 28–9, 133–7
        bandaging, 134
        causes, 135–6
        compression treatment, 134
        conditions causing, 135–6
        surgical treatment, 134–5
Venography, 126
Venotonic drugs, 136–7
Vertical banded gastroplasty (VBG), 97–8, 101

W

Web sites for evidence-based medicine, 30
Whipple's procedure, 14

X

Xoma, 58